black,
pregnant
and
loving it

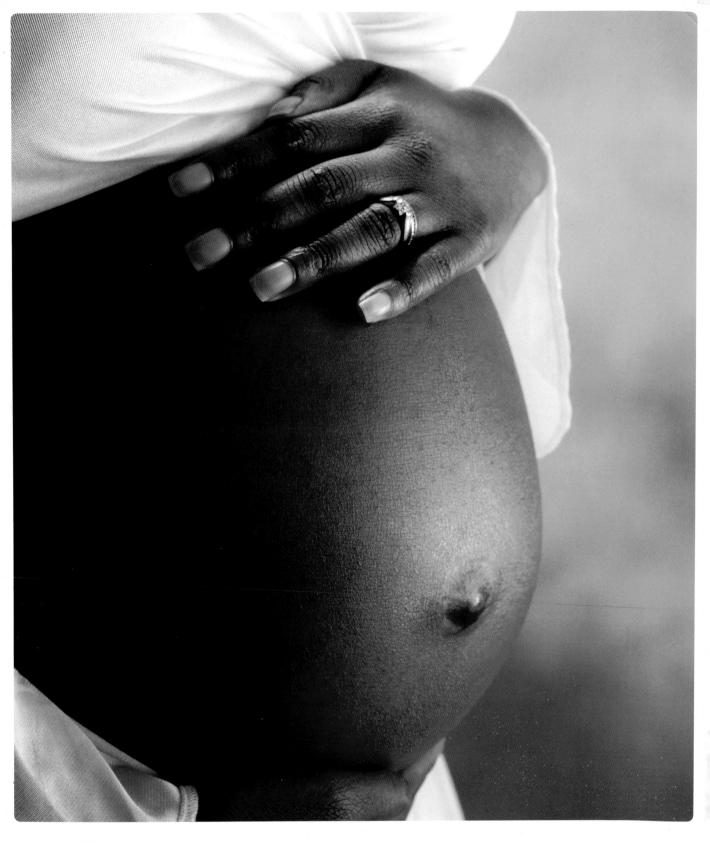

black, pregnant and loving it

the comprehensive pregnancy guide for today's woman of color

yvette allen-campbell and
suzanne greenidge-hewitt, MD

PAGE STREET
PUBLISHING CO.

PAGE STREET
PUBLISHING CO.

First published in 2016 by
Page Street Publishing Co.
27 Congress Street, Suite 105
Salem, MA 01970
www.pagestreetpublishing.com

Distributed by Macmillan, sales in Canada by The Canadian Manda Group.

19 18 17 16 1 2 3 4 5

ISBN-13: 9781624143151
ISBN-10: 1624143156

Library of Congress Control Number: 2016934575

Cover and book design by Page Street Publishing Co.
Cover image from Getty Images
Photography from iStock on pages 2, 6, 40, 52, 56, 66, 88, 95, 96, 104, 108, 113, 116, 121, 123, 130, 132, 136, 145, 149, 159, 154, 159, 165, 169, 173, 177 and 180
Photography from Getty Images on pages 10, 16, 18, 20, 24, 28, 32, 43, 80, 86, 90, 93, 105, 110, 111, 115, 118, 122, 126, 131, 139, 142, 146, 151, 155, 166, 174, 182, 186, 189, 194, 204 and 206
Photo editing on pages 88, 104, 113, 121, 130, 145, 154, 165 and 173 by Alexis A. Caudle

Printed and bound in China

Page Street is proud to be a member of 1% for the Planet. Members donate one percent of their sales to one or more of the over 1,500 environmental and sustainability charities across the globe who participate in this program.

Suzanne: I would like to dedicate this book to my grandparents, Edna Greenidge and Lawson Greenidge.

Yvette: I would like to dedicate this book to all of the little brown faces heading to schools across the country.

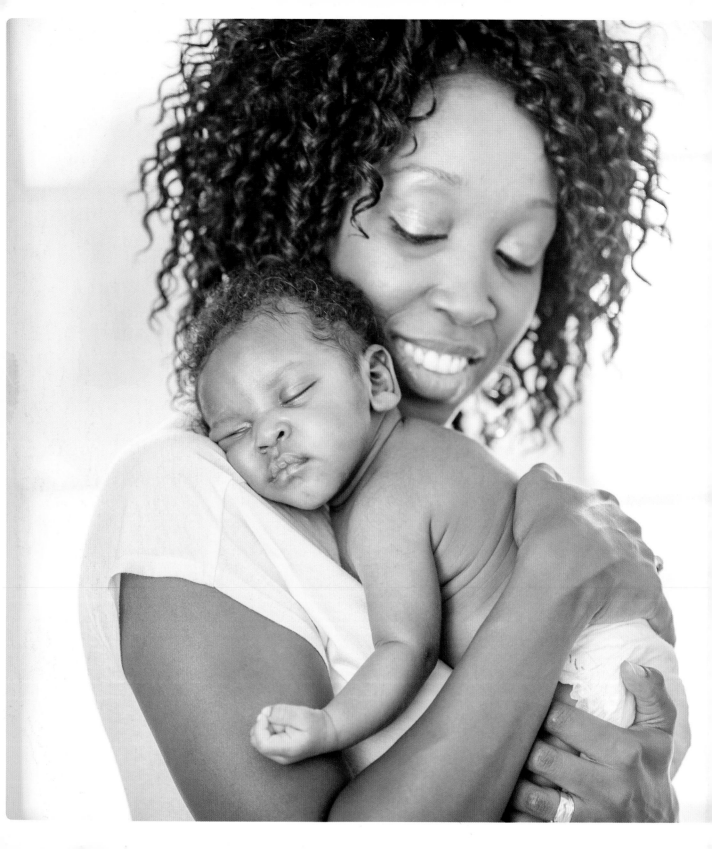

Part II
Your Pregnancy Month by Month — 87

Part III

The World Has One More Chance for Improvement: A Beautiful Black Baby Is Born! — 181

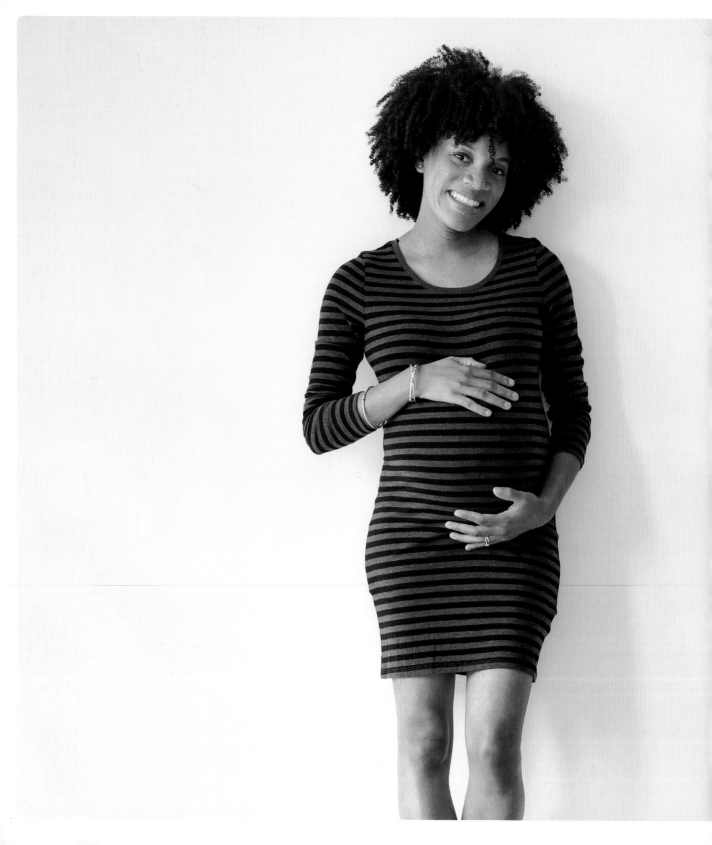

Why a Pregnancy Book Just for Us? Because It's Us! Beautiful Us!

Let's face it, ladies. It can be hard living in a culture that equates beauty with long, flowing hair and a rail-thin body, especially when you're the total opposite. That's why we validate and affirm ourselves. Reading a book that echoes just how beautiful you are during one of the most natural and vulnerable times in your life is a gift. This book is a gift, as is the birth of a baby into our society. We all get one more chance for improvement. Women should be celebrated and feel good about showing their beautiful pregnant bodies, and that includes black women.

We want and need to connect to a group that best matches who we are. Researchers have found that people showed greater brain activity when viewing faces belonging to their own racial group than when gazing at faces of a different race. We all have a strong social need to belong, and that's why we buy *Essence* and *Ebony* magazines.

Whether you have just found out you are pregnant or are planning to start a family, one thing is for sure: you are holding the right book in your hands. Unlike any other pregnancy book, this one includes month-by-month illustrations of a beautiful African American mom-to-be. But that is just the icing on the cake. In clear, nonthreatening language, we lay out all of the most authoritative and up-to-date information you need and want as you make preparations for your new baby. There is nothing as reassuring as having answers at hand for all of the questions that arise. We've done all we can to inform and reassure even the most anxious parents as well as childbirth "veterans" ready for their second or third babies.

A Message from Yvette

I spent nineteen years writing *Black, Pregnant and Loving It*. My career in education gave me one impetus for the book. In 1997, I was the principal of a private school, having spent the previous ten years in the New York City Public School System as a speech teacher, supervisor of speech teachers and assistant principal. It was during those times that I came face-to-face with the reality that an alarming number of African American children, especially boys, were being placed in special education programs. I had great concerns for the trajectory of these children's lives. Aside from some of the more obvious variables, such as systemic discrimination and cultural insensitivity, I wanted to know the differences, if any, in the development of white children and black children.

As I traced the development of specific skills in the two groups, I learned that many critical developmental milestones occur prenatally, before children are even born. Most alarming was that the "gap" started in the womb for many, with a disproportionate number of black children behind the curve. In 2000, twice as many black infants were born with low birth weight (developmentally delayed) than white infants, and three times as many black women died of complications of pregnancy and delivery than white women.

Armed with this information, I wanted to know what was on the market to inform pregnant women of the significance of this time in child development. On my trips to local bookstores, I discovered reams and reams of books on the topic. I found myself drawn to the pictures of the women with their huge bellies, almost in disbelief. None of the books showed pictures of pregnant sisters. None really spoke to me. Most of the books were clearly aimed at white women. When I read statements such as, "Your skin will become pink or reddened," I couldn't help but wonder what that meant for me. We shouldn't have to accept white women as the standard by which all women are measured; especially when our situations and outcomes can be vastly different. It was obvious that there was a void in the market when it came to informing and celebrating the pregnant African American woman.

I just couldn't live with that! Not only were black babies and black women experiencing serious health problems at a disproportionate rate, but the available information wasn't even written for us. So in 2000, I sought out the expertise of an experienced, highly regarded black obstetrician/gynecologist who happened to be working tirelessly at Harlem Hospital in New York City, Suzanne Greenidge-Hewitt, MD FACOG (fellow of the American College of Obstetricians and Gynecologists). Harlem Hospital at that time had over 5,000 deliveries per year with the majority being African American infants. Dr. Suzanne Greenidge-Hewitt and I began to write *Black, Pregnant and Loving It* in an attempt to respond to the unacceptable number of black women and black babies experiencing adverse pregnancy and childbirth outcomes. We finally completed the book and brought it into the world, a long gestation period, to be sure, but worth every bit of the time and effort it has taken to make the book all that it is meant to be.

Unfortunately, not a lot has changed since we started writing the book in 2000. Black children and their pregnant moms are still experiencing more than their fair share of difficulties and deficits during this precious time in their development. Dr. Greenidge-Hewitt has done her part caring for this vulnerable group. After a 26-year career in obstetrics and gynecology, becoming a board-certified obstetrician and gynecologist, laparoscopic/robotic gynecological surgeon, the founder and CEO of Woman to Woman OB/GYN and an avid spokesperson for women's reproductive health, she can proudly proclaim the healthy delivery of over 15,000 babies in her career. Although there are now a couple of books on the market aimed specifically at black women, none of them follow and illustrate the process of pregnancy and childbirth in the comprehensive and visual way that we do in *Black, Pregnant and Loving It*.

Everyone wants to identify with an image that they find desirable. *Black, Pregnant and Loving It* provides that opportunity; presenting realistic images and critically important information for the woman of color. My 30 years as an educator and my extensive research into the subject (with the help of Dr. Greenidge-Hewitt) make us uniquely qualified to bring this much-needed book into the world.

So our intentions are clear: we want you to be healthy, feel amazingly beautiful and honored to be pregnant. We want your babies to be strong and ultimately able to thrive in our society. To help make that happen, we explain how one of your first jobs as Mommy is to take care of business, such as the business of selecting the person who will help you deliver your baby. You will be presented with all of the different types of health-care providers that are available for you and their educational backgrounds. The message here is that you deserve the most competent, respectful and caring professional working for you and your baby. Don't settle for anything less. Use the information to make well-informed decisions for your growing family.

You will also be encouraged to modify your diet if it should need some tweaking. And for most of us, it usually does. There is no better time to become slightly more health conscious than when subjecting your unborn baby to whatever it is you are putting into your body. We offer explanations of what you will need for good health, and then back up the information with actual meals that are low in fat and salt yet still great-tasting.

Want to talk about sex? We do. Because although it's a little different during pregnancy, the physical contact that represents love is still very necessary to the pregnant woman and expecting dad. The more you know about what works sexually and sensually, the less worried and more loving you are likely to be.

Changes, changes, changes occur for 9 months, and we explain them all. From your hair to the mucous plug that keeps the baby inside of you, your body transforms in one heck of a way. The photographs of our beautiful brown-skinned models help represent the physical changes you will experience. We try to capture it all for you with words and photos!

You will also gain some understanding of that man of yours, thanks to a recurring section in the book called "Your Pregnancy & Your Man." Step-by-step we help you navigate those issues that can cause stress between you and your honey during your pregnancy. It's important in general, and especially as African Americans, to honor the bond you create when you put another human being on this earth. Statistics support that children being reared by both parents together do better in school than those who are reared by single parents. So as you embark on this journey of parenthood with your loved one, commit to the long haul.

To lighten things up a little, we share snippets of what it was like for our great-great-grandmothers to be pregnant. They made it work; we're testimony to it. Plus, there is always something precious to learn from our elders.

Going through labor and giving birth are some of the most anxiety-ridden experiences in a woman's life, and our objective is to get you through the process. Information truly is power, and the more you know, the more empowered you will be. So soak it all in and you won't feel so out of control during the big event. Don't get us wrong, there will be discomfort. But when you understand and expect it, you can flow better with it. And after all is said and done, you'll be able to stare lovingly at that gorgeous little brown face.

This is the beginning of the next chapter in your life: parenting the African American child. Although child development is not race specific, raising a black child in America does require special considerations. We offer food for thought as an educator and doctor for maximizing the health, safety and intelligence of your gift to our society.

Our appendices are chock-full of information as well. Sometimes taking the time to focus on little details just for you can generate your feelings of worthiness. That is certainly one of the missions of *Black, Pregnant and Loving It*. We want to provide for you because you are certainly worth it. The extras in the back of the book are resources that you might or might not need. You may find yourself in need of government assistance during this vulnerable time of your life, and that's okay. The assistance is there to ensure well-being for you, your child and your family when you are in need. In line with our unwavering dedication to you, Appendix A encourages you to structure a plan for economic independence. Without a clear way out of government support, there looms a threat of dependency, financial and psychological, for some women. We're not having that. Women are too valuable to get lost, so we hope that you can make your needs short-term. Just as when you make any kind of change in your life—career, relationship or health—there are steps you can take to get yourself moving in a productive direction. The key words are *moving* and *productive*, and we're behind you all the way.

The Prenatal Appointment Schedule Worksheet in Appendix B serves as a great way to collect personal monthly data during your prenatal visits with your health-care provider. Use it to jot down your questions and answers.

Appendix C offers you a snapshot of how state-based rights and protections for pregnant women and new parents compare to federal standards like FMLA, the Pregnancy Discrimination Act and Break Time for Nursing Mothers.

There is a lot to be said about pregnancy for black women, and we tried to cover it all. Our sole goal is for you and your baby to have the best chance for a healthy outcome and a prosperous life. Then we can finally say, after a decade and a half, "mission accomplished."

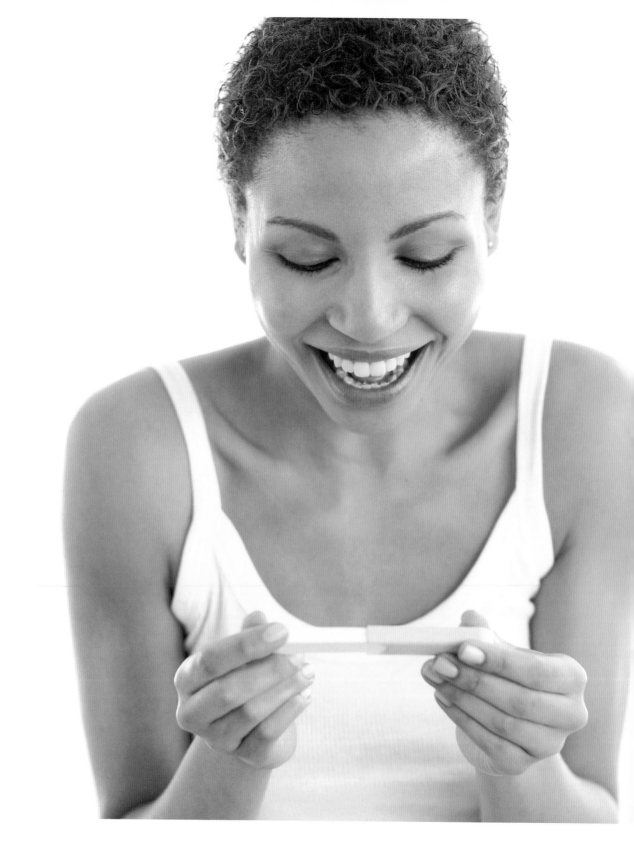

PART I

Getting Ready for Baby
"Me, as mommy? Sounds great!"

What a great feeling it is to be able to feel good about being a mommy, because for many of us the thought of pregnancy can be overwhelming. Whether you have dreamed about and planned for a pregnancy for many years in your head and in your heart or the news has taken you by surprise, take it from us: no matter what happens, you are in just the right place.

We have learned over many years that when we flow positively with our realities, we are more likely to live in peace and harmony. What a wonderful way of living our lives—wouldn't it be great if it came in a pill form? Simply take two pills with a glass of water in the morning and you've got yourself a day of peace and harmony! It's a nice fantasy, but in all seriousness, there is a lot to be said for maintaining a positive attitude and simply smiling.

Flowing with your new reality—you are going to bring a human being into the world—means doing some serious planning. It also calls for affirming and strengthening your relationship with the person with whom you created this new life.

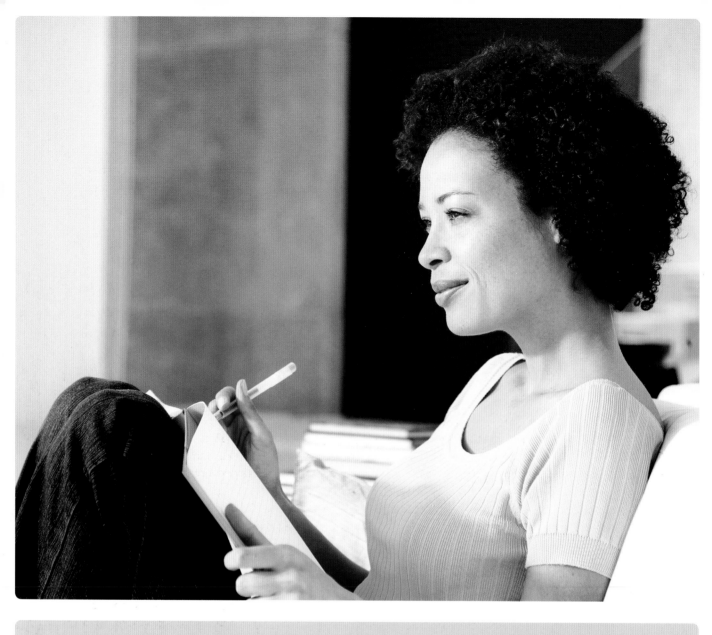

— CHAPTER 1 —

Planning Ahead

Becoming a mother will radically change your life as you know it, most likely for the better. If you're planning to stay home with your baby, the pattern of your everyday life will change dramatically. If you choose to resume your career, at the end of a day's work you have that gorgeous little face to come home to. No matter what happens during your day, you are always going to be the most important person in the world to your baby.

But the changes in your life after childbirth can wait. First, let's talk about the profound changes that occur during the course of your pregnancy. They are tremendous, and the sooner you begin to plan for them, the easier it will be later. This chapter tackles the first big decisions you must make.

Selecting a Doctor or Nurse-Midwife

"Who will help me deliver my baby?"

Next to your partner, your doctor or midwife is the most important person in your pregnancy. The person who provides you with care and helps you deliver your baby will have a big impact on your overall experience, so it is important that you feel very good and confident about your choice. Determining the most suitable medical partner for you and your baby is probably your first major decision as Mommy—and the same answer isn't right for everyone.

It's up to you to figure out what's right for you, your partner and your unborn baby—and that involves asking questions. A good place to start is by asking friends and relatives for recommendations of doctors and nurse-midwives with whom they've had good experiences. At the same time, it's important for you and your partner to talk to each other. Share your feelings and beliefs about pregnancy and childbirth. Perhaps you agree that you'll feel safer with a conventional medical birth in a hospital, in which case you will probably be happiest with a medical doctor. If a natural approach is more your style, you may want to consider a nurse-midwife. If you're not sure of what's right for you because you don't know enough about the options that are available, please turn to the Planning Baby's Birthday section of Chapter 9, "The Fifth Month." That section is dedicated to explaining in detail the choices for managing labor and childbirth.

Make sure that you can come to a consensus about the kind of care you are looking for. You certainly want your lives to be in the hands of competent, experienced professionals, which has no bearing on race or ethnicity. However, in most instances, it is an added bonus for women to have a doctor of color. It's no secret that people who share similar values, experiences and cultural patterns feel more comfortable with each other. So if you do a little research or get a reference for a highly regarded black practitioner, you and your family may be the beneficiaries of a skilled provider who engenders a sense of comfort and familiarity to you.

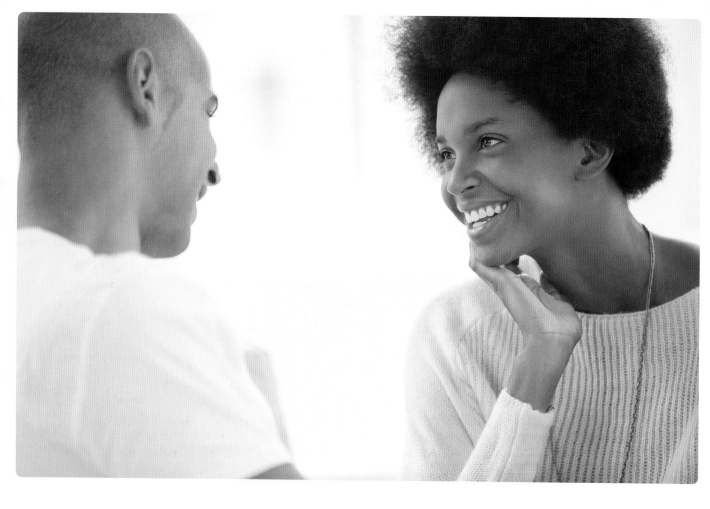

Either way you should meet in person with your prospective practitioner. This initial interview is your opportunity to determine whether you feel a good connection and sense of trust. Is this the person you want to care for you and help you deliver your baby? Big on your assessment checklist should be whether or not you and the practitioner share similar pregnancy and childbirth philosophies. So take some time to really think about and envision your baby's birthday. What type of experience would you like your family to have, assuming all is well and you can have it your way. Does this match the kind of care this professional provides?

You will also want to get a sense of whether or not your personalities are compatible and whether you can communicate easily and clearly. Be prepared to ask questions of yourself as well as of the practitioner, and make yourself thoroughly familiar with the potential birth site. Listen carefully and try to be realistic, since no relationships are absolutely perfect.

Here are some questions to ask any potential practitioner:

- What are your beliefs regarding natural childbirth? Be ready to share your interpretation of what natural childbirth is to you, since the practitioner may ask you to describe how you envision proceeding through a natural childbirth. (Review the natural childbirth section in Chapter 9 for more information.)

- Under what conditions will you decide to bring on labor with medications rather than allow me to continue naturally? *This question is important because if you're planning to take an active role in managing your labor and delivery, then you'll need to know when your practitioner will step in and make a unilateral decision regarding the progress of your labor. A good answer to this question is "when the risks of proceeding naturally outweigh the benefits." You can ask for an example of the conditions that would make inducing labor safer. This information can help you better understand what to expect during labor.*

- Will I be able to walk around freely during labor? *Some practitioners will monitor you and the baby continuously throughout the entire labor while you remain in bed; others will allow you to walk around free of monitors as long as you report back periodically for monitoring. Some health-care providers now have the technology to allow you to move around freely while being monitored.*

- Under what conditions do you find it necessary to use tools such as forceps or vacuums to move the baby through the birth canal? *Practitioners vary in their protocols for using these tools. In general, however, if a woman gets too tired to push during labor, or if the baby is in distress, her doctor may use forceps or a vacuum to assist her.*

- Do you routinely perform episiotomies? (Pronounced *eh-pih-ZEE-ot-uh-meez*, a cut between the vaginal opening and the anus that allows more room for the vaginal delivery of your baby.) *If you feel strongly about avoiding an episiotomy, make sure to inform your provider.*

Here are some questions to ask the practitioner about the site where the birth will take place:

- Does the site allow more than one person in the labor room? *If you wish to have family members or friends present during your labor or delivery, you need to be aware of the hospital's policies.*

- Does the site have features such as birthing rooms? (Birthing rooms are hospital rooms that look like cozy bedrooms, where you can labor, deliver and recover all in one place.)

- Does it have rooming-in policies that allow the baby and the father to stay with the mother?

- What is the level of the newborn nursery? *Level one is for healthy newborn babies. Level two is for babies that require special care. Special care is usually designated for babies who are born at 32 weeks and up. Levels three and four are the neonatal intensive care units.*

- Do they allow a family member in the labor, delivery and operating rooms even during cesarean births?
- Would I have to keep my legs in stirrups during delivery? *There are different positions a woman can move into during labor and delivery. The more conventional positions involve stirrups, but some women prefer other positions, such as squatting. If the freedom to move into various positions is important to you, a practitioner who tends to be less conventional may be the best choice.*

Once you've asked the prospective practitioner these questions, and any others that may be important to you, you'll want to think about his or her answers. Here are a few questions you might want to ask yourself in order to make an informed assessment:

- Does this person seem to be a good listener and a careful explainer?
- Will he or she take my concerns about the emotional aspects of pregnancy seriously?

Be aware that if your pregnancy is considered to be high risk, your choices are limited. Conditions that might put you into the high-risk category include chronic hypertension, diabetes or a history of a premature delivery. Obviously the top priority in a high-risk pregnancy is ensuring the health of mother and child, and other preferences might have to take a backseat. The doctor you like the most or the birthing techniques that are most comfortable or convenient for you may not be the best choices for a healthy delivery.

If you're unsure whether you are high risk or not, you'll probably find out during your first prenatal visit with your health-care provider. That appointment will probably include a detailed discussion about your medical and obstetrical histories. This information you provide will help your doctor determine whether or not you are at high risk for complications.

We don't want to alarm you, but you should be aware that unanticipated complications can arise as early as your first month of pregnancy, or you might sail through the first trimester and develop complications later. If your doctor determines that you are in the high-risk category, he or she may refer you to a perinatologist (maternal fetal medicine specialist [MFM]), a doctor who specializes in high-risk pregnancies.

The Selection Criteria

When developing your criteria for selecting a doctor or midwife, here are a few things you should consider.

COMPETENCE IS KEY

Competence is the major requirement of a health-care professional. In medicine, competence is associated with formal training, board certification, hospital affiliations and good references.

How can you be sure the person you want to select has the right training? Here's a primer on the different types of practitioners who deal with pregnancy and what to look for in each:

- A physician specializing in obstetrics and gynecology (OB/GYN) is either a doctor of medicine (MD) or a doctor of osteopathic medicine (DO) who has received special training that includes four years of residency in a hospital. He or she has then gone on to become board certified in obstetrics and gynecology. Any doctor you select should be certified by the American Board of Obstetrics and Gynecology. Don't assume that all the doctors you interview are board certified because it isn't mandatory everywhere. Don't be afraid to ask about this during your initial interview—it is a perfectly reasonable question.

- A perinatologist, also called a maternal fetal medicine specialist (MFM), deals specifically with high-risk pregnancies. This specialist completes the same four years of residency as an OB/GYN but then goes on to complete another three years of training as a fellow of perinatology. He or she then goes on to be board certified in perinatology. You'll want a perinatologist to manage your pregnancy if you have diabetes, hypertension or any other disorder that puts you at risk for having complications during your pregnancy. Depending upon your circumstances, a perinatologist may be your only doctor until you deliver, or he or she may co-manage with your general OB/GYN, in which case you will see them both.

- A family practitioner has had several years of training in primary care, including obstetrics, after receiving an MD. If you and your family have been using a family practitioner over a relatively long period of time, then he or she has the benefit of knowing you well and understanding your particular health (and emotional) dynamics. This can be a great advantage, presuming that you are not experiencing a high-risk pregnancy.

- A certified nurse-midwife (CNM) is a licensed independent health-care provider with the ability to prescribe medication in all 50 states, if needed. These professionals often care for women throughout their reproductive life span, and have a special emphasis on pregnancy, childbirth and gynecologic and reproductive health. CNMs are certified by the American Midwifery Certification Board (AMCB). Prior to taking the national certification examination, they must graduate from a nurse-midwifery education program accredited by ACNM. Eligibility to enter such a program requires a bachelor's degree from an accredited college or university along with an RN license in most instances. Most CNMs work in clinics, private offices, hospitals or birthing centers. They monitor the soon-to-be-mother's health and that of her unborn baby during pregnancy through regular prenatal visits. Due to their vast knowledge and training in the field of obstetrics, they should be able to address any of your questions and concerns. CNMs assist women during labor and delivery and are trained and experienced in postpartum and normal newborn care, in addition to routine gynecological care. But what's most special about this group of health-care providers is that they pride themselves on offering women a compassionate partnership with individualized methods of care. The certified midwifery profession includes certified midwives (CM) and certified professional midwives (CPM). Each title carries distinctive credentials. For more information consult midwife.org or the AMCB at www.amcbmidwife.org.

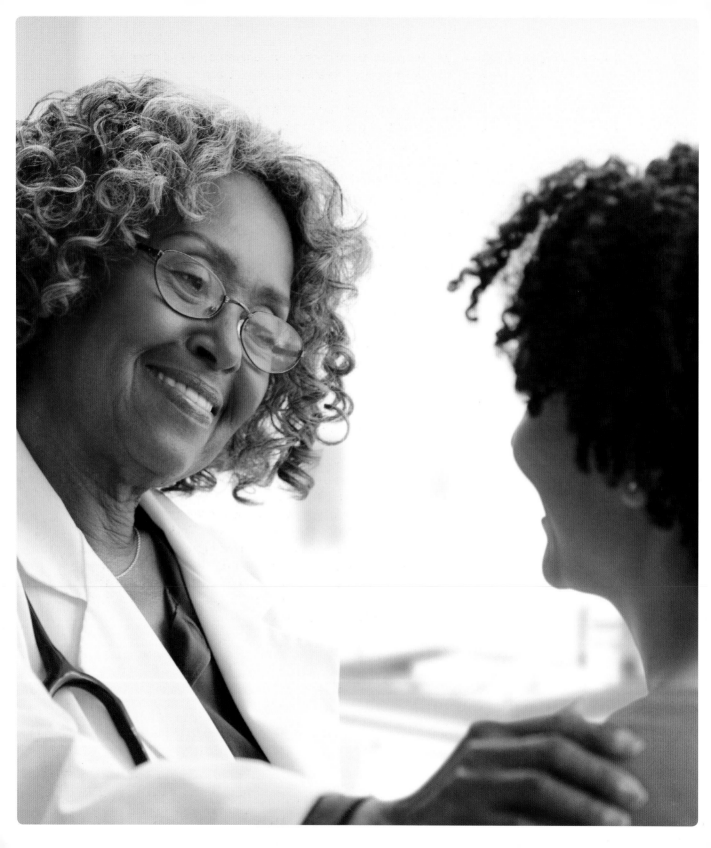

Another indicator of competency is the doctor's affiliations with various hospitals, known as his or her "privileges." For example, a doctor might be affiliated with a teaching hospital or a community hospital. He or she may admit patients only to the hospitals with which he or she is affiliated. Some people prefer doctors who have affiliations with teaching hospitals because they feel the doctor may be more up to date with the latest technology and research. Make no mistake about it, hospitals matter. You do want to check out the reputation of a hospital, the quality and level of its neonatal intensive care unit (NICU), whether it has a center for high-risk pregnancies and certainly its health insurance policies. The federal government's website www.medicare.gov/hospitalcompare allows you to find a hospital by location or name and compare it with up to two other hospitals within a certain mile radius. The *U.S. News and World Report* provides an annual ranking of the best hospitals nationally and regionally. The Leapfrog Group grades hospitals from A to F on how safe they keep their patients from errors, injuries, accidents and infections. So check out the hospitals with which your doctor is affiliated because when you choose a doctor, you are also choosing a hospital.

In the world of medicine, formal training is undeniably important, along with board certification and hospital affiliations. But don't underestimate the value of good old-fashioned word of mouth. A health-care provider's competence is also reflected in what his or her patients say to their girlfriends, coworkers, neighbors and family members. Listen carefully to anyone who wants to recommend a doctor, and tell them you want complete honesty about their experiences with their providers.

Some last words on competence: a doctor or midwife of your own ethnic background may have a better understanding of your culture, and consequently may be more sensitive to your fears and beliefs. He or she may also more easily recognize and monitor important environmental and genetic factors that relate to you. A case in point: I once consulted a white dermatologist about a recurring scalp problem I was having. During our appointment, I told her about the hair touch-ups I got every six weeks. She immediately concluded that the chemicals in these treatments were probably my problem and told me to stop the treatments! I'm sure you can imagine that this was an impractical recommendation—impossible, really—as it would be for many black women. At the time, I considered it an insensitive and worthless recommendation, but I suppose it could be chalked up to cultural ignorance. In any case, I would have been better off consulting a doctor more familiar with the concerns black women have about their hair. A practioner of color might have recognized the importance of touch-ups to black woman and provided medical treatment options that work with the chemicals in those hair care products.

LOOK FOR RESPECT

Mutual respect should exist at all times between you and your doctor or midwife. Although the person you choose will have expertise in a certain area, he or she should always be willing to listen to your opinions, concerns and fears, and address them in a professional manner. You deserve nothing less.

A respectful, trusting relationship with your health-care provider will also make it easier for you to disclose any important information about your life that could affect your pregnancy. For example, during your first prenatal visit, your doctor may ask you about your personal habits, such as whether you drink alcohol, smoke cigarettes or indulge in any illegal or controlled substances. You may question why your health-care provider has to pry into these matters and may even be tempted to give incorrect information. Don't do that. Find the right practitioner for your family now—so you won't feel the need to undermine the process by withholding important information from her or him. This isn't about passing moral judgment; it's about increasing your odds of having a healthy pregnancy and baby. Remember, though, that if at any point during your relationship with your provider you feel uncomfortable or believe you are being judged inappropriately, by all means discuss this with her or him, and if necessary look for someone else. Health-care practitioners work for you—they are not doing you a favor. There is absolutely no good reason why you should accept substandard service. A positive, trusting relationship with your health-care professional is key to your well-being during this momentous time.

Although we all know it, we would be remiss if we didn't make the statement that alcohol, cigarettes and recreational drugs can destroy your body's ability to create a healthy environment for your baby to grow. If these habits are a part of your reality, it's extremely important that you tell your doctor. She or he may be able to assist you in abstaining from these substances during your pregnancy. Your doctor will also want to monitor your baby more closely, since drinking, smoking and drug use can lead to low birth weight and other developmental problems. Forgive the sermon if this isn't your issue—but we're sure you know that it is an important one within our community. You, too, probably cringe when you see so many of our young people unable to compete and thrive in mainstream America.

It's illegal for any health-care organization to discriminate against anyone by race, creed, color, sexual preference, religion or national origin. If you feel you have been the object of discrimination, or if you have any other problem with the care and services you have received, take your complaint to your provider or hospital and request a written response if you desire. Hospitals have a patient's bill of rights (feel free to ask for a copy at any time) that delineates what patients are entitled to. It holds the hospital accountable for providing patients with quality service, and entitles you to complain without fear of retaliation and to receive an answer in writing. If you are not satisfied with a hospital's response you can complain to your state's Department of Health.

Taking Care of Business

"How am I going to juggle pregnancy and work?"

Your pregnancy should be one of the most special times of your life and that of your partner. Not only is a child being made in your likeness and from your love, which alone is reason enough for celebration, but society at large is being given another chance for improvement through the existence of a new human being. When you consider pregnancy in this light, it would make sense for our society to protect and support our childbearing population. Unfortunately, this is not always the case, so you must be sure to take steps to protect yourself and your baby. The first step in doing this is to understand your rights and entitlements.

Public Policy and Your Rights

"Work with me here."

In the United States only three laws exist that address pregnancy and support for new families: the Pregnancy Discrimination Act, the Family and Medical Leave Act (FMLA) and Break Time for Nursing Mothers.

The Pregnancy Discrimination Act of 1978 was the first law that addressed pregnancy and support for working women. It was created to protect women from being fired, denied promotions or demoted because of pregnancy. The law mandates that companies with more than fifteen employees treat pregnancy like any other medical disability. That may sound like a good thing, but the law leaves a lot to be desired in terms of protecting the rights of pregnant employees.

First of all, pregnancy is not a disability and shouldn't be referred to as one. This type of inappropriate labeling perpetuates the thinking that once a woman becomes pregnant she can no longer fulfill her responsibilities at work. Secondly, this act only ensures that pregnant women receive the same benefits as other employees with similar inabilities to work, and these benefits can be inadequate in covering pregnancy and maternity.

FMLA, passed in 1993, requires employers to offer employees 12 weeks of unpaid, job-protected leave for the birth or adoption of a child; to care for a newborn; or to care for a spouse, child or parent with an illness serious enough to prevent the employee from working. Dads are eligible for this leave, and they can go on leave before the baby is born. Unless you are having a problematic pregnancy, however, you'll probably want to save all of your time for after the birth of your baby. (Trust us, it goes by quickly!)

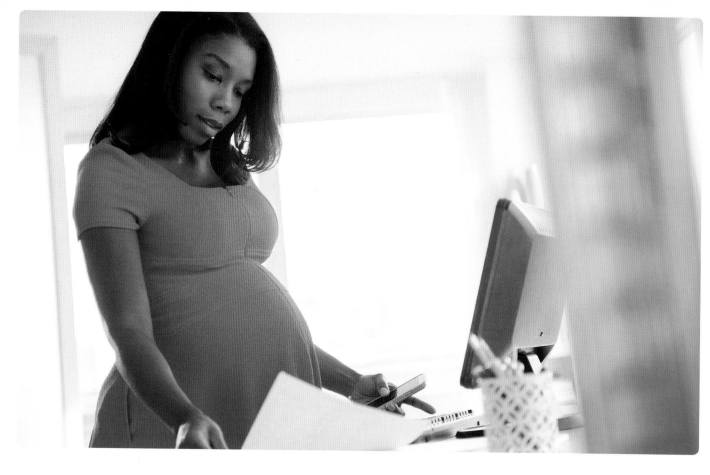

Be aware that there are certain limitations on eligibility for this leave. The act is enforceable only for employers with 50 or more employees and exempts the highest-paid 10 percent of them. The employee must have worked for his or her current employer for at least 12 months and worked for at least 1,250 hours. Either parent may take the leave as long as she or he meets the above requirements, but the leave must be taken within the first 12 months after the baby's birth (or placement, in case of adoption).

An employee is required to request this leave 30 days before it is to begin, if possible. In the case of a premature delivery, the leave should still be honored. During the twelve-week leave period, all employee benefits provided to regular employees are to be continued at the employer's expense. These include group life insurance, health insurance, disability insurance, sick leave, annual leave, educational benefits and pension benefits. Accruals for seniority and certain other benefits do not have to be provided during the leave.

The law says that an employee who returns from leave "must be restored by the employer to the position of employment held by the employee when the leave commenced" or to a position of the same pay, benefits and conditions of employment.

We've given you an overview here, but due to the complexity and significance of this law, our best advice is to do your research and consult with those who thoroughly understand it to determine how it will affect you. Don't overlook your own colleagues when seeking advice. There may be a woman in your company who has already taken advantage of FMLA. She will probably be extremely knowledgeable about it and may be able to guide you in the right direction.

Break Time for Nursing Mothers exists because of the 2010 health-care reform law that gives women returning to work after having a baby the "right to pump" for one year after giving birth. Nursing mothers protected by this law are entitled to reasonable break times and a private place within the workplace to pump breast milk. This law is restricted, however, to women who are paid hourly or those who are eligible for overtime.

Understand Your Employee Benefits

Fortunately, many companies provide maternity benefits that exceed the requirements of the law. The most important thing that you can do to make sure you receive what you are entitled to is to thoroughly understand what's included in the benefits program you receive from your employer. Find out about insurance policies (such as temporary disability insurance), maternity leave, sick leave and medical disability leave that your employer may offer. Your Personnel or Human Resources Department should be able to provide you with all of the information you require. You should also be able to find answers to your questions in your employee manual or handbook—but make sure you have the most updated version. If anything seems unclear, or if you are uncertain about how something applies to your situation, ask.

MATERNITY LEAVE

Maternity leave is an umbrella term that refers to two types of time away from your job to care for your baby: maternity leave and family leave.

Maternity disability or medical leave is meant to provide you with time away from work after the birth of your baby to recuperate and care for your newborn. On average, companies provide women with six weeks off after childbirth. Be aware that most companies don't provide *paid* leave, and they don't have to. For that reason, women often use any accrued sick days they have (paid days off) before starting the clock on their unpaid maternity leave.

Another important fact is that as of this writing, maternity leave does not extend to the father or adoptive parents (though, again, some companies choose to offer "paternity leave" and extend these benefits to adopting couples).

The other type of maternity leave is family leave, which you are entitled to under FMLA as described previously.

PATERNITY LEAVE

In the United States, there is no law that mandates that companies provide paid paternity leave. That leaves you and your partner at the mercy of his employer in granting him time away from work to care for your newborn baby. We are impressed to report that many companies now acknowledge the importance of this time for fathers and include provisions for paternity leave in their benefits program. Your man's Personnel or Human Resources Department is the best source of information on the subject. If paternity leave is not included in his benefits program, he can do what most men in his position do and use accrued vacation or personal days to spend time at home with you and the baby.

Just to be clear: he *is* entitled to FMLA, but this is not paid leave. It simply protects his job and benefits should he choose to spend significant time with you and your newborn.

The good news is that some states provide more than the modest protection provided by the three federal laws for working parents. We've included a brief summary of each state's provisions in Appendix C. It's just a quick snapshot of what each state offers beyond the Pregnancy Discrimination Act, FMLA and Break Time for Nursing Mothers. It may not be conclusive, so still do your homework in scoping out all that you are entitled to receive.

Getting the facts about your rights and entitlements is incredibly important for you and your growing family. Speaking with colleagues who have been in your shoes can be just as informative, if not more. You may not find the answers to the little nuances of juggling pregnancy and work in an employee handbook. Here are some questions you may want to ask a coworker who has gone through the process:

- What did you say to your boss when you told him or her about your pregnancy and plans for maternity leave?
- How did your boss and colleagues respond when you told them about your pregnancy and plans for maternity leave?
- What forms did you fill out and where did you get them?

- How much time did you take off?
- How did you structure your leave?
- What arrangements did you make to have your responsibilities covered during your absence?
- How did you transition back to work? Who did you notify when it was time to return to work?
- Is there anything that you would do differently now, looking back on your maternity leave?

If you're still interested in doing your own research on issues concerning leave from work, any local or regional office of the US Department of Labor's Wage and Hour Division will be able to provide you with more information.

Well, Mom, this is it! You've taken the first of many steps in ensuring your child's well-being. You can now focus on giving your baby a solid foundation in life by providing a loving, nurturing, healthy experience in the womb.

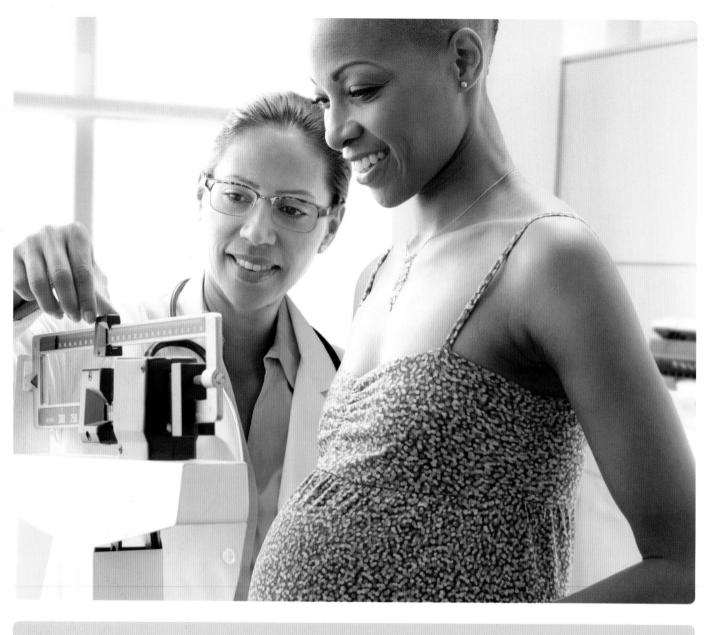

— CHAPTER 2 —

That All-Important Diet

Everyone seems to have an opinion or philosophy about conception, pregnancy and childbirth. Many describe it as a miracle, others say it's purely physical and most everyone agrees that pregnancy requires people who are knowledgeable. Mom, let's face it, as amazing as you are, you have little control over the miracle of birth. The little one inside of you pretty much takes over the physical aspects of pregnancy, leaving you with owning and using the information needed to bring forth life into the world. This chapter is dedicated to providing you with all of the information you need to eat right and maintain a healthy body for you and your precious son or daughter.

Weight During Pregnancy

Your unborn baby's body grows from the nutrients it receives from you. So undoubtedly you will gain extra weight to support your baby. How much you will need to gain depends on your pre-pregnancy weight and your body mass index (BMI).

Your Body Mass Index

Measuring BMI is a relatively new approach to understanding weight and its connection to your overall health. BMI is a measure of your body fat based on your height and weight. This is such an important health factor that the American College of Obstetricians and Gynecologists (ACOG) recommends that a BMI be recorded for all women at their first prenatal visit. A woman entering pregnancy at an unhealthy weight or high BMI increases the risk of a number of disorders during pregnancy, including hypertension and diabetes. Your doctor will need to be aware of these risk factors so that she can try to prevent the onset of the disorder or be prepared to manage it should you start to experience symptoms.

This is a subject that should touch a nerve with a good number of us since over half of all black women, 56 percent, have high BMIs, placing them in the obese category. If you have three friends, chances are that two of you are obese. This book exists to celebrate and inform the pregnant black woman. We wouldn't be sincere if we said we weren't worried about that statistic.

The BMI table below explains the categories of weight based on a woman's BMI number.

BMI	CATEGORY
< (less than) 18.5	Underweight
18.5–24.9	Normal Weight
25–29.9	Overweight
30–34.9	Obese Class I
35–39.9	Obese Class II
40 and above	Obese Class III

So what's the plan for the pregnant woman who has a high BMI? In view of associated risks, ACOG recommends the following:

- Overweight women (BMI of 25 to 29.9) are advised to gain no more than 15 to 25 pounds during pregnancy.
- Obese women (BMI of 30 and higher) should gain 11 to 20 pounds during pregnancy.
- Obese women should be offered and should consider nutrition consultation and are encouraged to follow an exercise program.
- All women should be screened for gestational diabetes at the initial prenatal visit with repeated screening later in the pregnancy if the results are negative.
- Women with a BMI of 35 or greater who have pre-existing medical conditions, such as hypertension or diabetes, may benefit from a cardiac evaluation.

Gaining Weight

The American College of Obstetrics and Gynecologists recommends that women who begin pregnancy at a healthy weight (not underweight and not overweight) gain 25 to 35 pounds during the entire pregnancy. This weight gain should be spread across the entire three trimesters; about 5 pounds in the first trimester and about 1 pound every week for the rest of the pregnancy. That may sound like a lot of weight, but even the most disciplined woman can fall into the thinking of "well, I'm eating for two so I can have another slice . . ." and before you know it, 25 pounds turns into 45 pounds easily.

It is sometimes recommended that the underweight woman gain more weight during pregnancy. The exact amount of weight gain for an underweight woman is based upon her individual needs. If you are either underweight, overweight or obese, your health-care practitioner will more than likely put you on an individualized weight-control plan.

Alcohol Consumption

Before we get into all the nutrients that you need to consume for a healthy pregnancy, let's set the record straight about alcohol intake. There is always some confusion about whether or not it's permissible for a pregnant woman to drink alcohol. We're calling it: no they can't. Alcohol goes into the bloodstream and passes through the umbilical cord to the unborn baby. So the wine, martini or beer that you drink, your unborn baby takes in as well. Children exposed to alcohol in utero are at risk for growth deficiencies, intellectual deficiencies, facial deformities and central nervous system impairments. There is no safe time in a pregnancy for a woman to drink alcohol. An unborn baby's brain is developing throughout pregnancy and can be affected by alcohol at any time. The ACOG as well as the Centers for Disease Control and Prevention both agree that there is no amount of alcohol that is considered safe to drink at any time during a woman's pregnancy.

Now, let's get real for a minute. Just because you are pregnant doesn't mean you're immune to life's hassles, those almost unbearable situations that often make a glass of wine at the end of the day your best comeback. Instead of drinking wine, do something else. Put on your favorite song, turn the volume up and dance, or get comfortable on the sofa and watch your favorite movie again. For me it's *The Best Man Holiday*; Suzanne can't get enough of *Dream Girls*.

If you have already consumed some amount of alcohol, most likely prior to you even knowing you were pregnant, don't fret over it. Worrying about the past can take up a lot of emotional energy and there is nothing you can do about it. You can make sure that from this moment on you will consume a variety of nutrients that will help keep your mind and your body strong and free of ailments.

What Your Body Needs for Good Health

In general, most of the nutrients required for a healthy pregnancy can be met by eating ordinary, readily available food. Since many women don't get enough specific nutrients, especially iron and folic acid, vitamins are often prescribed to meet those recommended dietary allowances (RDA).

We emphasize the importance of good nutrition for your unborn baby's development for very good reasons—it's his or her lifeline. In this chapter we explain in detail the variety of nutrients you and your baby will need for good health. To make this information more useful, we also provide the United States Department of Agriculture's (USDA's) recommended servings of healthy food from each food group for pregnant women.

Energy

Human energy is seen in the movement of our bodies through muscle action and in the heat that our bodies produce. Energy comes from the metabolism of the food we eat and is obviously a requirement for all human beings. During pregnancy your energy requirements are increased. You need more energy to produce new body mass for both you and your developing baby. You'll also need more energy to move your extra body weight. The RDA of energy is expressed in calories, and pregnant women require 2,300 to 2,400 calories a day, which is about 275 to 300 calories more than the pre-pregnancy requirements. But that's really not a lot since merely drinking four glasses of skim milk (360 calories) and taking the required extra serving of protein can push you over your limit. Be very selective about what you eat! Remember, even though you're eating for you and your unborn baby, he or she is extremely small. Any additional calories beyond 2,400 daily are excessive and ultimately can create a challenge for you when you're trying to get back into your skinny jeans.

Protein

You and your baby will also need protein. Protein is what builds muscles, blood, skin, hair, nails and your baby's internal organs. It's composed of large combinations of amino acids. The human body needs 22 of these amino acids for proper growth, development and maintenance of health. They're extremely important in pregnancy to build the cells of a new baby.

The body can synthesize (make by using the elements within our bodies) 14 of these amino acids; however, we must get the remaining eight essential amino acids from the foods we eat. Certain foods called complete proteins can provide us with all eight essential amino acids. They are meat, poultry, fish, eggs, milk and milk products such as yogurt and cheese. The RDA of protein for the average pregnant woman is 74 grams a day.

Vitamins

Vitamins are organic compounds (that which comes from living organisms, like plants) that everyone needs for normal body functioning. Our bodies can't create vitamins, so we have to get them from what we eat or from dietary supplements. No one food contains all the vitamins we need, which is why a varied diet is so important for us. One of the ways vitamins are classified is according to their ability to dissolve in fat or water. It's important to know which vitamins are fat-soluble and which are water-soluble. Water-soluble vitamins dissolve in water, which makes it relatively easy for excessive amounts of it to leave our bodies through urine. Fat-soluble vitamins, on the other hand, dissolve in fat, causing them to linger in the body longer.

FAT-SOLUBLE VITAMINS

During pregnancy your requirements for fat-soluble vitamins increase. In many cases, maintaining a well-balanced diet will adequately provide all the fat-soluble vitamins you and your baby need. The fat-soluble vitamins are:

- **Vitamin A.** During pregnancy vitamin A is needed for fetal development and for the formulation of colostrum (mother's first breast milk). Too much or not enough vitamin A has been known to produce birth defects in infants. The RDA of vitamin A during pregnancy is 770 retinol equivalents. A retinol equivalent is the measurement used for quantifying the value of vitamin A. Eating fresh vegetables like carrots, cantaloupe, spinach and collard greens regularly should provide you with an adequate amount of vitamin A. Here's a good tip for spotting foods rich in vitamin A: they are usually red, orange, yellow or dark green, so watermelon, sweet potato and macaroni and cheese are also significant sources of vitamin A.
- **Vitamin D.** Pregnant women need vitamin D to promote a positive calcium balance. Be careful when taking a vitamin D supplement, though, since too much vitamin D can cause toxicity in the mother and the unborn baby. The RDA for vitamin D during pregnancy is 10 micrograms (mcg). Food sources for vitamin D include fortified milk, egg yolks, sardines, shrimp and tuna.

- **Vitamin E.** Being an antioxidant, vitamin E protects our cells from damage. It also helps our body's digestion and our ability to respond to stress. The RDA for vitamin E during pregnancy is 15 mg. Consuming vegetable oils, peanuts, tomatoes, ready-to-eat cereals, sunflower seeds, turnip greens, egg yolks and whole grains can supply us with the needed amount of this essential nutrient.

- **Vitamin K.** We can get vitamin K from bacterial metabolism in our intestines and from leafy green vegetables such as greens and spinach. The amount of vitamin K in an ordinary diet is usually enough for pregnancy. The RDA of vitamin K during pregnancy is 90 mcg. Good sources of vitamin K are egg yolks, collard greens, kale, spinach, turnip greens and broccoli. This vitamin plays a role in ensuring that the blood of both mother and unborn baby clots sufficiently. After delivery, vitamin K injections are routinely given to newborns to help prevent bleeding problems.

WATER-SOLUBLE VITAMINS

Water-soluble vitamins dissolve in water as opposed to fat, and they include the B-complex vitamins and vitamin C.

- B-complex vitamins include B_1 (thiamine), B_2 (riboflavin), niacin, B_6, folic acid, biotin, B_{12} and pantothenic acid. They're all pretty much interdependent of each other in carrying out their specific functions in the body.

- Thiamine, riboflavin and niacin play an important role in your ability to produce energy. You certainly don't want to run out of energy now, especially as you proceed in your pregnancy. The RDA of thiamine during pregnancy is 1.4 mg. The RDA for riboflavin during pregnancy is 1.4 mg, and for niacin it's 18 mg. Good sources of thiamine, riboflavin and niacin are whole grains, legumes, pork, milk, cheese, lean meats, soybeans, yogurt, ready-to-eat cereals and green leafy vegetables.

- Vitamin B_6 aids the body's ability to metabolize amino acids. It also works with niacin in energy production. B_6 can be found in whole grains, soy flour, organ meats, wheat germ, prune juice, bananas, chickpeas, mushrooms and potatoes. The RDA of vitamin B_6 during pregnancy is 1.9 mg.

- Biotin aids in your use of proteins and other B-complex vitamins. Rich sources are egg yolks, cheddar cheese, beef liver, peanuts, cauliflower, avocado and mushrooms. Its RDA during pregnancy is 30 mg.

- Folic acid is part of the B-complex group and works with vitamin B_{12} and vitamin C in the breakdown and use of proteins. You need more than twice as much folic acid as a nonpregnant woman. Since the typical American diet doesn't contain enough of this vitamin, you can easily become deficient. A diet with too little folic acid may lead to poor development of the fetus and placenta, which is why supplements for folic acid are routinely given to pregnant women. Ask your doctor about a folic acid supplement at your first prenatal visit, since it's important to begin taking folic acid as soon as you know you're pregnant. Folic acid and vitamin B_{12} play an important role in the development of your baby's nervous system. Providers recommend that women take 180 mcg of folic acid prior to getting pregnant and 400 mcg while pregnant. The RDA of vitamin B_{12} during pregnancy is 2.6 mcg. Ready-to-eat cereals, lentils, black eyed-peas, spinach and beef are some sources of folic acid. Vitamin B_{12} on the other hand is more readily available in cooked crabs, cooked clams, ready-to-eat cereal, beef and lamb.

- Vitamin C. Although the need for vitamin C increases during pregnancy to 85 mg per day, this increase is often entirely met through your diet alone. Vitamin C is not stored in the body, and therefore you need to get some every day. Vitamin C is found in many of the foods we eat. Citrus fruits such as oranges and grapefruits, and vegetables such as collard greens and turnip greens are excellent sources. A lack of vitamin C can cause common problems such as nosebleeds and bleeding gums. You may find relief from these discomforts by increasing your daily intake.

Minerals

You and your baby must get an adequate amount of minerals during pregnancy. They're just as important as your protein and vitamin supply. Minerals are inorganic substances (that are not from living structures) that play a vital role in regulating many body functions. There are many that you need, but the most essential minerals during pregnancy are:

- **Iron.** Your iron needs to double during pregnancy. Your baby will take what he or she needs, causing your body's iron demands to increase. Your body requires 27 mg of iron daily to adequately meet your baby's needs as well as yours. You need this much iron because it helps your blood and your baby's blood carry oxygen from your lungs to your cells, and carbon dioxide from your cells back to your lungs. It's highly unlikely that you'll meet these iron requirements by diet alone since the typical American diet is deficient in iron. You can ensure that you get enough by taking iron supplements alone or as part of prenatal multivitamins. If you are anemic, ask your provider if you should take both iron supplements and multivitamins. If you are not anemic, prenatal multivitamins and an adequate diet will provide sufficient iron. Although years ago iron supplements had a bad reputation for causing constipation, newer formulations of the supplement are easier on your digestive system. Good food sources of iron include beef, duck, soybeans, oysters, dried fruit, egg yolks, cooked clams, chicken, lentils and kidney beans.

- **Calcium.** Every day you and your unborn baby need about 1,000 mg of calcium. It's needed for the growth of the baby's bones and teeth. For you, taking in more calcium helps replenish calcium deficiency brought on by pregnancy. Although it's believed that many women can fulfill their calcium requirements through an appropriate diet that contains milk and dairy products, this is not the case for the women who cannot digest these foods. Difficulty digesting dairy products is called lactose intolerance. Many African Americans have this problem, which causes gas, diarrhea and abdominal pain. If digesting dairy products, including milk, is a problem for you, you can try lactose-reduced milk and nondairy foods that are high in calcium such as canned sardines, salmon with the bones, dark leafy green vegetables and black-eyed peas. It may ultimately be necessary for you to take calcium supplements or antacids. Tums is an antacid that is not only a good source of calcium, but it's also considered safe during pregnancy. By the way, taking calcium supplements has also been linked to reducing preeclampsia (see Chapter 3 for details on this condition).

Vitamin and Mineral Supplements

Most women take vitamin and mineral supplements during pregnancy, but they are not a substitute for a healthy, wholesome diet. In fact, eating an ordinary, well-balanced diet is a far better way for you and your baby to get almost all of the vitamins and minerals you need. Iron and folic acid are the only exceptions.

For most of us, though, supplemental vitamins are necessary. So do some research and talk to your provider. Understand that an over-the-counter prenatal vitamin may provide 100 percent of the RDA for one vitamin or mineral but not enough for another. Additionally, know that in the vitamin supplement world, 100 percent isn't always the best and most desirable. For example, a prenatal vitamin can provide you with more than 100 percent of the RDA for vitamin A. So a pregnant woman who takes this kind of supplement and eats a normal diet could be consuming excessive amounts of vitamin A, which can be toxic in high doses. We know all of this can sound confusing, so the best thing that you can do is consult with your health-care practitioner when in doubt.

Please, Someone, Translate This into Real-Life for Me!

So now you're probably thinking that you know how important energy, protein, vitamins and minerals are for you and the baby, but what does it all mean for you from day to day and meal to meal?

First of all, it helps to know that the USDA has developed a food guide that categorizes all of the food we eat according to the type of food it is and how much of it the human body requires. The USDA's website has a section on health and nutrition for pregnant and breastfeeding women, which you can find at www.choosemyplate.gov/moms-pregnancy-breastfeeding. It can be a good resource for you regarding your dietary needs.

Next, to make all of the nutritional requirements that we've talked about more realistic, we will list common food items in their respective food group, and give you the number of servings that you and your baby need daily from each food group to keep healthy. The food groups are divided into dairy, protein, vegetables, fruits and grains.

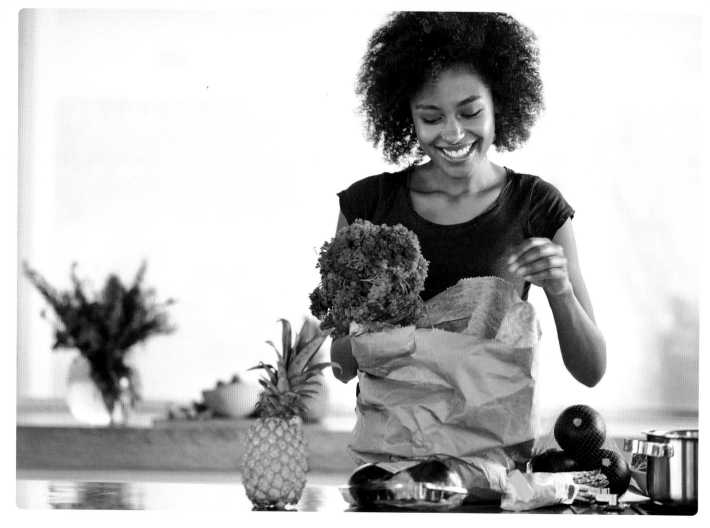

Dairy

MILK & CHEESE

Eat three to four servings from this food group every day! One cup is the equivalent of one serving. Good examples of food from this group include:

- Fat-free or low-fat yogurt
- Fat-free milk (skim milk)
- Low-fat milk (1 percent milk)
- Calcium-fortified soymilk
- Reduced-fat or low-fat Lactaid milk

Protein

MEAT, POULTRY, FISH, EGGS & BEANS

Eat two to three servings from this food group every day! Good examples of food from this group include:

- Beans and peas (such as red kidney beans, black-eyed peas, lentils and chickpeas)
- Nuts and seeds
- Lean beef, lamb and pork
- Crab, mussels and oysters
- Salmon, trout and sardines

Do not eat fish with excessive amounts of mercury in it, such as shark, swordfish, tilefish and king mackerel. Mercury can be harmful to the brain and nervous system if a person consumes too much of it. Although there are trace amounts of mercury in nearly all fish, the amounts are generally so small they are harmless to us. The exceptions are the four fish listed above. You should also be aware that white tuna (albacore) contains much less mercury than the four fish to avoid, but it contains three times as much mercury as light tuna. The US Food and Drug Administration (FDA) recommends that you limit your intake of white tuna (albacore) to no more than six ounces per week.

Vegetables

Eat two to three servings from this food group a day! Good examples of food from this group include:

- Collard greens
- Kale
- Spinach
- Carrots
- Sweet potatoes
- Pumpkin

All of the above vegetables are great sources of vitamin A and potassium. If you opt for canned vegetables, make sure you choose a low-sodium or no-salt-added brand.

Fruits

Eat three to six servings from this food group a day! Good examples of food from this group include:

- Cantaloupe
- Oranges
- Red or pink grapefruit
- Mangoes
- Honeydew melons
- Bananas
- Apricots
- 100 percent juice orange juice or prune juice

If you opt for canned fruit, make sure you choose a brand with fruit canned in 100 percent fruit juice or water rather than syrup.

Grains

BREAD, CEREAL, RICE & PASTA

Eat two to three servings from this food group every day! Good examples of food from this group include:

- Oatmeal
- Brown rice
- Popcorn, with little to no added salt or butter
- Wheat bread
- Whole wheat cereal flakes
- Macaroni
- Spaghetti

There are so many kinds of cereal. Make sure you choose one made from whole grains and fortified with iron and folic acid.

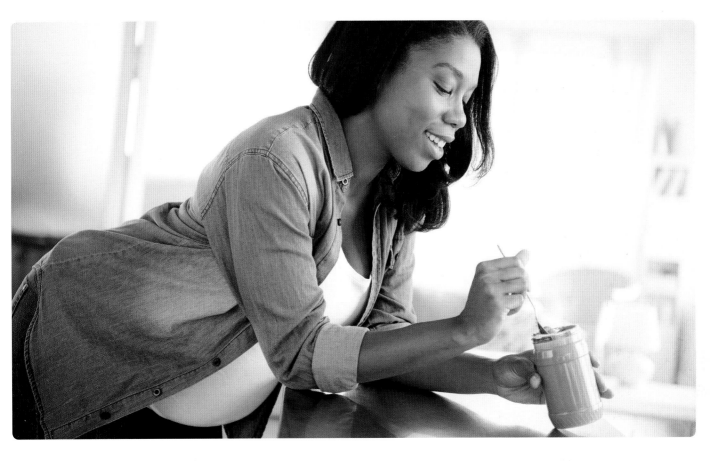

It Has to Taste Like Something!: Healthier Soul Food Recipes

Although we know that our foods, our very *soul* foods, are cultural and a part of our identity, we must be honest and admit that the way many of us prepare some of our foods can be harmful to us—pregnant or not. And of course this matters more than ever when there's a baby on board.

Excessive amounts of salt and fat in our diets can take a toll on our bodies. Hypertension, preeclampsia (see Chapter 3 for more about that condition) and excessive weight from fatty calories can have their way with us. But let's also keep it real: we know that if the food doesn't taste good, we're not going to eat it! We need a balance. So here are some traditional soul food recipes that have been revamped to cut the fat, salt and cholesterol without sacrificing the flavor. We enlisted executive chef Denzil P. Richards, culinary graduate of the New York Restaurant School, to prepare them especially for you!

Tasty Main Courses

Brown Stew Chicken

Yield: 4 servings

Stews are great all-in-one meals, and the bonus is the leftovers. Somehow, there is always enough to nibble on for a few days, which can be a godsend when your pregnancy has got you dragging.

1 whole chicken, cut into serving portions, skin removed

Salt or salt substitute (such as Mrs. Dash) and pepper to taste

1 tsp fresh thyme, chopped fine

½ cup (25 g) scallions, chopped fine

1 tsp garlic powder

¼ tsp allspice

1 tsp onion powder

2 medium Yukon Gold potatoes

2 cups (470 ml) low-sodium chicken stock, divided

3 carrots, roughly chopped

2 medium onions, roughly chopped

2 medium-sized roma tomatoes, roughly chopped

1 green bell pepper, roughly chopped

2 tbsp (30 g) tomato sauce

4 tbsp (60 ml) olive oil

Season the chicken with salt or salt substitute and pepper, thyme, scallions, garlic powder, allspice and onion powder. Cover and place in the refrigerator overnight.

Bring 1 quart (960 ml) of water to a boil and add the potatoes. Boil for 15 to 20 minutes, until fork tender.

Drain the potatoes and let cool, then puree in a food processor with ½ cup (118 ml) of chicken stock.

Combine the roughly chopped vegetables and tomato sauce in a 2-quart (2-L) saucepan with 2 cups (480 ml) of water and the remaining chicken stock. Simmer for approximately 30 minutes.

Remove the chicken from the refrigerator. Place a 2-quart (2-L) saucepan on medium heat. Pour the olive oil in the pan. As soon as the oil is hot, sauté the chicken, for 5–8 minutes, turning frequently until it's lightly brown on all sides.

Transfer the cooked chicken to the saucepan with vegetables, and allow it to simmer for an additional 35 minutes. Gradually add the pureed potato to the saucepan until you achieve the desired thickness, and allow the stew to cook for an additional 15 minutes until done.

Sautéed Red Snapper or Monk Fish with Wild Herbs

Yield: 2 servings

If you're looking for a tasty, healthful meal that you can serve up in no time, a fish dish will never let you down. The problem with fish is that many of us are so used to deep-frying it to get that great fish smell and taste. Here's a recipe that cuts the fat because you're sautéing the fish in olive oil only briefly, then letting it bake—still tasty without adding much preparation time. It's delicious, healthy and fast to make.

2 lb (1 kg) red snapper or monk fish

Salt or salt substitute (such as Mrs. Dash) and pepper to taste

1 dash lemon pepper

1 tbsp (15 ml) olive oil, divided

¼ cup (38 g) chopped onions

1 cup (240 ml) low-sodium chicken stock

1 whole scallion

¼ cup (43 g) chopped green pepper

¼ cup (40 g) chopped tomato

1 tsp thyme

1 tbsp (14 g) margarine

Preheat the oven to 350°F (180°C).

Season the fish with salt or salt substitute, pepper and lemon pepper to your taste.

Sauté the fish in olive oil for about 5 minutes per side until it's golden brown.

Place the fish on a baking sheet and into the oven to continue to cook for 10 to 15 minutes.

While the fish is baking, prepare the sauce in a sauté pan.

Add 1 teaspoon olive oil and the onions, and cook on medium heat for 1 minute until just translucent. Add the chicken stock, scallion, green pepper, tomato, thyme and margarine, plus salt and pepper to taste, and simmer for 10 minutes.

Remove the fish from the oven and place on a serving dish. Pour the sauce over the fish and serve.

Rosemary Roast Turkey

Yield: 4 to 5 servings

As we all try to cut back a little on how much red meat we eat, we're challenged to come up with creative and varied poultry dishes. Rosemary Roast Turkey is a nice alternative—it's not just for Thanksgiving anymore!

1 (6-lb [3-kg]) turkey

1 tsp onion powder

1 tsp granulated garlic—not garlic powder

Salt or salt substitute (such as Mrs. Dash) and pepper to taste

2 carrots, roughly chopped

2 stalks celery, roughly chopped

1 clove garlic, minced

2 medium onions, roughly chopped

2 tbsp (2 g) fresh rosemary, roughly chopped

Preheat the oven to 375°F (190°C).

Remove the giblets and neck from the turkey, and rinse the turkey with cold water, inside and out.

Sprinkle the onion powder and granulated garlic inside and outside of the bird.

Season with salt or salt substitute and pepper inside and outside.

Mix the carrots, celery, minced garlic, onion and 1 tablespoon (1 g) of the rosemary. Place this mixture inside the turkey, being careful not to overstuff the bird. Truss the turkey by tying the legs and wings in place. Place in the refrigerator for 1 hour.

Sprinkle the remainder of the rosemary over the bird and put in the oven, uncovered.

Roast for approximately 3 hours, basting periodically with pan drippings.

Use a meat thermometer to check the internal temperature of the breast. When it reaches 165°F (74°C), it's ready to come out. Rest for 10 minutes before slicing.

Sautéed Sesame Seed Medallion Pork Loin in Honey Glaze Sauce

Yield: 4 servings

Maybe you've chosen to cut pork out of your diet because of its high salt and fat content—or because your religious beliefs forbid eating it. But many African Americans continue to eat and enjoy pork because of its rich flavor and the fact that it's a staple in many of our cherished soul food dishes. If you love pork as much as we do, keep in mind that fresh pork, rather than cured, is a much healthier choice.

For this tasty dish, Denzil has chosen the loin because it's the softest cut of the meat with a minimal amount of fat. He uses olive oil because it is lower in saturated fat than many other fats and oils—but be careful because it burns very quickly.

---

2 lb (908 g) fresh pork loin, boneless, cut into medallions

Salt and pepper to taste

¼ cup (60 ml) olive oil

1½ tsp (7 ml) sesame oil

1 rosemary stem

1 oz (28 g) sesame seeds

HONEY GLAZE SAUCE

1 tbsp (15 ml) olive oil

2 large red bell peppers

½ onion

1 clove garlic

2 tsp (10 ml) honey

1 cup (240 ml) low-sodium chicken stock

1 tsp paprika

1 tsp ground cumin

Salt or salt substitute (such as Mrs. Dash) and pepper to taste

Preheat the oven to 350°F (180°C).

Season the pork loin medallions with a small amount salt and as much pepper as you like. Combine ¼ cup (60 ml) olive oil, 1½ teaspoons (7 ml) sesame oil and 1 rosemary stem, and add the medallions. Marinate overnight.

Remove the medallions from the marinade and coat both sides with sesame seeds, pressing to make a solid, even coating.

Put the remaining oil in a sauté pan and heat on the highest setting. Sauté the pork for 3 minutes on each side, making sure it is just cooked through.

Lay the medallions on a sheet pan and place in the oven to complete cooking, approximately 10 to 15 minutes.

To make the glaze, preheat the oven to 375°F (190°C). Slightly coat a cookie sheet with olive oil.

Place the whole peppers on the sheet and bake for 20 to 25 minutes.

Allow the peppers to cool in an airtight container for 15 minutes. Remove the outer skin, inner core and seeds, and then slice.

In a food processor, puree the onion, garlic and bell peppers.

In a saucepan, combine the bell pepper mixture with honey, chicken stock, paprika and cumin. Simmer over medium heat for approximately 10 minutes.

Add salt or salt substitute and pepper to taste. Pour over the cooked pork. This glaze works well over chicken, too.

Beans and Rice

It's hard to go wrong with a bean dish. Beans are inexpensive yet high in protein, making them the perfect alternative to meat, poultry or fish. Here are two easy options we think you'll enjoy.

Red Beans and Rice

Yield: 4 servings

1 cup (200 g) dry red kidney beans

¾ cup (180 ml) coconut milk

1 tsp garlic powder

¼ tsp nutmeg

Pinch of allspice

1 whole scallion

½ tsp thyme

2 cups (470 ml) low-sodium chicken stock

1½ cups (316 g) rice

Soak the beans overnight in a container with enough water to cover them completely.

Bring 4 cups (960 ml) of water to a boil and add the beans. Boil vigorously for about 40 minutes, until fork tender.

Add the coconut milk, garlic, nutmeg, allspice, scallion, thyme and chicken stock. Return to a boil, then turn down the heat and simmer for approximately 10 minutes.

Add the rice, cover the pot and set on low flame so the liquid reduces slowly and the rice is cooked. This should take about 25 minutes. Check frequently and add more water if necessary. The rice is ready when all of the water is absorbed.

Beans and Yellow Rice

Yield: 4 servings

1 cup (240 ml) low-sodium chicken stock

1 cup (200 g) dry black beans (soaked overnight to speed cooking)

1 tsp onion powder

1 tsp granulated garlic

1 tbsp (14 g) low-fat butter

1 tsp curry powder

Salt or salt substitute (such as Mrs. Dash) and pepper to taste

2 oz (57 g) margarine

1 cup (210 g) rice

1 tsp fresh basil, finely chopped

Fresh parsley, chopped, for garnish (optional)

Bring the chicken stock and 2 cups (480 ml) of water to a boil and cook the soaked beans until soft, about 40 minutes.

Add the onion powder, garlic and butter, and continue to simmer for 15 more minutes.

In another pot, bring 1 quart (960 ml) of water, curry powder, salt or salt substitute, pepper and margarine to a boil and add the white rice. Cook for about 25 minutes, until the rice is fork tender. Fold in the basil.

Divide the rice into bowls and top with black beans. Garnish with parsley if you wish.

Scrumptious Side Dish

Potato Salad

Yield: 4 servings

A good home-cooked soul food meal just isn't complete without potato salad. In this healthier version, Denzil has left the potato skins on because of all the rich nutrients they contain. Egg whites, rather than whole eggs, reduce the cholesterol tally—and of course the low-fat mayo has the same effect.

It may not be Mom's recipe, but we think you'll like it!

2 whole Yukon Gold Potatoes

3 eggs

¼ cup (38 g) green peas

¼ cup (55 g) low-fat mayonnaise

1 tbsp (16 g) Dijon mustard

1 tbsp (15 g) minced shallots

1 tsp lemon juice

¼ tsp onion powder

1 pinch white pepper (black pepper is fine as long as you're OK with black specks in the potato salad)

Bring 1 quart (960 ml) of water to a boil, add the potatoes and cook for 15 to 20 minutes, until fork tender.

In another pot, boil the eggs for 13 minutes, then shock them in an ice water bath.

Boil the green peas in 1 quart (960 ml) of water for 20 minutes, drain.

Remove the shells from eggs, separate and discard the yolks.

Roughly chop the potatoes, then combine them with the green peas, mayonnaise, Dijon mustard, shallots, lemon juice and onion powder. Add in the egg whites and a pinch of white or black pepper as desired.

Dessert

All-Fruit Fruit Salad with Raspberry Syrup

Yield: 12 servings

What meal would be complete without something sweet? Nobody said you couldn't enjoy dessert, as long as you watch your portions—and that includes what happens in the kitchen when you're cleaning up!

8 cups (1 kg) raspberries, rinsed and drained

8 cups (1.6 kg) strawberries, rinsed, drained and halved

1 cup (144 g) blackberries, rinsed and drained

2 ruby-red grapefruit, peeled, seeded and sectioned

3 seedless (navel) oranges, peeled and sectioned

1 medium pineapple, peeled, cored and cut in chunks

1 cup (150 g) seedless grapes, rinsed and drained

1 small cantaloupe, peeled, seeded and cut in chunks

2 Granny Smith apples, peeled (if desired), cored and cut in chunks

1 Asian pear, peeled (if desired), cored and cut in chunks

1 banana, peeled and sliced

2 kiwifruit, peeled, seeded and cut in chunks

1 mango, peeled, seeded and cut in chunks

1 papaya, peeled, seeded and cut in chunks

2 tsp (6 g) dark brown sugar

4 mint leaves, shredded (optional)

Puree 6 cups (740 g) of raspberries and then 6 cups (1.2 kg) of strawberries, and then combine the two purees. Place the puree in a 1-gallon (4-L) saucepan and bring it to a boil. Reduce the heat to low and simmer until the mixture thickens.

Strain the mixture through a fine strainer, discard the solids and set aside the remainder to cool.

Combine all the remaining fruit and separate into 12 serving bowls. Sprinkle each fruit bowl with ½ teaspoon of dark brown sugar.

Drizzle approximately 2 teaspoons (10 ml) of the berry sauce over each fruit bowl.

If desired, garnish with shredded mint leaves. Serve at room temperature.

Healthy Breakfast Meals

Breakfast is the most important meal of the day, yet we can easily skip it as we rush out the door in the morning. Slow down and fuel your body the better way.

Old-Fashioned Oatmeal with Granola & Fresh Fruit

Yield: 4 servings.

This is a tastier version of a healthy breakfast meal that always hits the spot and will keep even a pregnant lady full until lunchtime.

2 cups (160 g) rolled oats

1 cup (237 ml) skim milk

1 tbsp (9 g) brown sugar

1 tbsp (7 g) nutmeg

1 tbsp (8 g) cinnamon

½ cup (61 g) granola

1 banana, peeled and sliced

1 cup (200 g) strawberries, rinsed, drained and halved

In a 2-quart (2-L) saucepan, stir together the rolled oats and 2 cups (480 ml) of water. Place on medium heat and simmer for about 8 minutes, until the oatmeal is tender.

Remove the pan from the heat and add milk, brown sugar, nutmeg and cinnamon.

Portion the oatmeal into 4 serving bowls. Sprinkle 2 teaspoons (10 g) of granola onto each one, and then add equal parts bananas and strawberries.

Egg White Vegetable Omelet

Yield: 2 servings

This dish should satisfy your egg craving without all the cholesterol.

1 red bell pepper, finely diced

1 green bell pepper, finely diced

½ medium white onion, finely diced

½ medium red onion, finely diced

1 scallion, finely chopped

1 tomato, finely diced

4 egg whites

Salt or salt substitute and pepper to taste

2 tsp (10 ml) olive oil

4 slices whole wheat or multigrain toast

Combine all the vegetables.

In a mixing bowl, whisk egg whites lightly, and then add a little salt and ground pepper to taste.

Place a large sauté pan on the stove over high heat. Allow the pan to become very hot, and then add the olive oil. When the oil is hot, pour the egg whites into the saucepan.

Immediately add the vegetables in the center of the saucepan, and use a spatula to fold the egg whites over the vegetables to create the omelet. Cook for 1½ minutes, flip once, and then remove it from the pan.

Serve with toast.

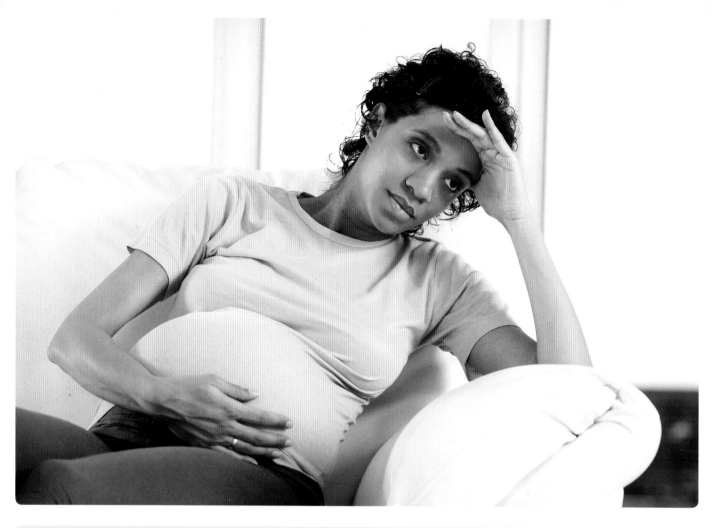

CHAPTER 3

Health Issues Common to Pregnant Black Women

The probability of black women experiencing certain disorders during pregnancy is as much as three times higher than it is for women from other ethnic groups. These disorders include preeclampsia, gestational diabetes and fibroids. We are also at a higher risk for premature labor. Explanations for these disparities are sometimes biological in nature and may involve hereditary factors, but in many cases there is not enough research to fully explain why a disorder disproportionately affects black women.

Undoubtedly, socioeconomic status and psychological state are contributors to our health outcomes. Sadly, a relatively large percentage of black women are physically or mentally unhealthy due to lifestyle factors, some of which are not in their control. But, particularly at this important time in life, all women should carefully monitor their health. So even if you are living a secure and healthy lifestyle, the information in this section is relevant—and extremely important. If you find yourself compromised by a disorder covered in this chapter, rest assured that you are not alone. Doctors have been battling these disorders for years. Unlike our ancestors, we can rely on modern medicine to secure our lives and the lives of our unborn children. If your pregnancy is proceeding as expected, thank God and feel free to skip this section.

Although hereditary factors and lifestyle can contribute to complications, pregnancy by itself can be problematic, as in the case of preeclampsia. Furthermore, pregnancy may cause changes to pre-existing conditions such as diabetes, hypertension and asthma, which can become real challenges to manage in a pregnant body.

We hate to dwell on the negative, but remember that knowledge is power. The information in this chapter is intended to help you make healthy decisions for you and your baby. At the end, we've included a worksheet that you can use to chart any medications you may need to take, the reasons for taking it, the dosage and the dates that you use it. Keeping a record of this information can be very useful for you and your doctor, and will provide a reference for future pregnancies as well.

Facing Our Problems Head-On!

The conditions we discuss here can really complicate our lives and throw us into emotional turmoil. If you have or develop a disorder during your pregnancy, our first piece of advice is to try to learn as much as possible about it, beginning with the summaries in this chapter. Our second suggestion is to try to view the situation as part of your unique existence, and that it has a purpose. Adversity can make us stronger, smarter, more sensitive and inspirational to others. And if it does, then we've done our best with what we've been given.

Hypertension Disorders of Pregnancy

"Did you take your pressure pills today?"

"All of a sudden I just couldn't fit my feet into my shoes!"

The most common medical complication of pregnancy is hypertension disorder. Most of us are all too familiar with this condition, either from firsthand experience or that of a relative or friend who battles it. It's hard to avoid, since 45 percent of black women age 20 and older have hypertension, compared with 27 percent of white women. Here's what you need to know about how hypertension relates to pregnancy.

The National High Blood Pressure Education Program Working Group on High Blood Pressure in Pregnancy has defined four categories of hypertension in pregnancy:

1. Chronic hypertension
2. Gestational hypertension
3. Preeclampsia
4. Preeclampsia superimposed on chronic hypertension

What Hypertension Is

Hypertension, another name for high blood pressure, exists when the force of your blood flow persistently pushes very hard against the walls of your arteries, causing damage to blood vessels. Throughout the day, it's normal for the intensity of this force to increase and decrease, but when it stays at an increased level, you have high blood pressure.

Blood pressure is measured using two numbers: the *systolic* and the *diastolic*. The systolic number reveals how hard your blood is pushing when your heart is pumping; the diastolic number tells you how hard your blood is pushing between heartbeats, when your heart is relaxed and filling with blood. Normal blood pressure for adults is somewhere within the range of 120 over 80 (120/80) with the systolic on top and diastolic on the bottom. Blood pressure in adults is considered high when readings are above 140/90. When your blood pressure is high and is pushing very hard against your artery walls, it starts to damage the heart, blood vessels and kidneys. This is why hypertension is a key risk factor for heart disease and a leading cause of death among African Americans.

One of the most dangerous characteristics of hypertension is that it can cause such life-threatening damage without presenting any symptoms that you can feel and would prompt you to seek medical attention. A disease or disorder that exists without symptoms is all too easy to ignore or deny. Particularly during pregnancy, failing to take the necessary precautions and to seek appropriate treatment can threaten the health of both mother and child.

Causes of hypertension include chronic kidney disease and thyroid disorders, although in most cases doctors can't identify an exact cause. When a specific cause cannot be found, hypertension is called "essential." A poor diet, obesity, family history and lack of exercise have all been identified as contributors to hypertension.

A major concern for the obstetrician caring for a pregnant woman with hypertension is ensuring that the baby is receiving an adequate amount of oxygen for optimal growth. When hypertension occurs during pregnancy, blood flow to the placenta decreases, causing a reduction in the baby's oxygen and nutrient supply. This can lead to premature separation of the placenta from the uterine wall (placenta abruptio, discussed later in this section). This can affect the development of the baby's organs, cells and body systems. If left untreated, not only can the baby be smaller, it can also lead to stillbirth. Doctors can determine or estimate the size of an unborn baby by measuring the mother's fundal height (how large her belly is growing) and looking at ultrasounds. An ultrasound is a test that uses safe sound waves to create images of your unborn baby.

Specific treatment for high blood pressure during pregnancy really depends on the patient's category of hypertension, discussed in more detail below. In general, however, care includes teaching the patient how to take and read her own blood pressure on a daily basis. Self-blood pressure readings are most accurate when taken after sitting or lying for a while.

Sleeping in a side-lying position may be recommended as a way to improve blood flow to the baby. This helps prevent the uterus from pressing on the major blood vessels of the mother's heart, thereby increasing blood flow to the uterus.

Blood pressure is highest when the mother is active. It's imperative to remember that it's the lack of oxygen to the placenta that is most dangerous to the baby. Since there are no drugs that increase blood flow to the placenta, bed rest may be recommended, along with doctor visits at least every two weeks, frequent ultrasounds to rule out fetal growth restrictions and the avoidance of excessive physical activity.

Maintaining a well-balanced diet and limiting salt intake are important to managing hypertension as well. Fresh and protein-rich foods and vitamins should replace processed and fatty foods whenever possible (see Chapter 2 for more on healthy eating). If blood pressure is under control before and during pregnancy, both mother and baby should thrive.

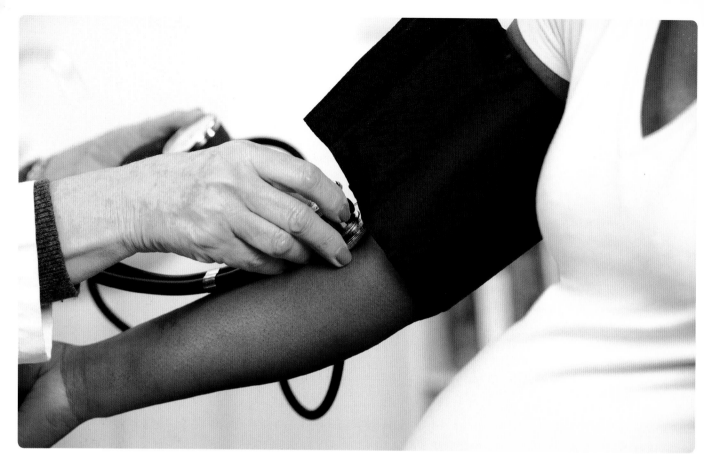

CHRONIC HYPERTENSION

Hypertension that starts in the first half of pregnancy—before 20 weeks—is usually considered to be chronic (an ongoing problem that can last for a lifetime). If it first occurs later in pregnancy, it's called gestational hypertension.

Chronic hypertension complicates just 6 to 8 percent of all pregnancies in the United States but can cause serious complications such as heart failure, kidney failure, stroke or eclampsia (seizures). We know it sounds scary, but keep in mind that relatively few pregnant women are affected by it to a profound degree. And keep in mind that just by choosing to read this book, you have demonstrated your commitment to becoming informed and staying healthy. You are already a great mom!

Stacy's Chronic Hypertension

Stacy was 36, an executive in the technology field, with two children ages 10 and 7 when she discovered she was 12 weeks pregnant. At her first prenatal care visit with her OB/GYN, her blood pressure reading was 155/95. She had a history of hypertension, which had been diagnosed 5 years earlier, well after her last pregnancy. She had taken blood pressure medication for a while, but had not taken any in the last 2 years. She never felt any of the symptoms of high blood pressure, such as headaches or vision problems.

Because Stacy's blood pressure was elevated, her obstetrician informed her that she might need to take medication during her pregnancy. He also referred her to a perinatologist for consultation. For the duration of her pregnancy, both doctors monitored Stacy's health carefully. As long as her blood pressure was under control, she was allowed to continue to work.

Although Stacy began her pregnancy with untreated hypertension, the care she received from her health-care team helped keep her healthy throughout her pregnancy. She also took an active role in her own health by checking her blood pressure at home every day and resting on her side whenever possible. She was able to maintain a healthy environment for her unborn baby, who was delivered full term, vaginally, weighing 6 pounds, 3 ounces. "Prince" Jordan, the only boy in the family, now gets a lot of doting attention from his older sisters.

TREATING CHRONIC HYPERTENSION DURING PREGNANCY

If you suffer from chronic hypertension—especially if you are not already under treatment for it—early prenatal care is critical to a healthy pregnancy. If you are diagnosed early, your obstetrician can develop an effective management plan that might include a referral to a perinatologist.

If you are contemplating pregnancy and you know you suffer from hypertension, be sure to discuss treatment options with your obstetrician prior to conception. Most women with mild to moderate chronic hypertension usually do well during pregnancy and do not require medication. However, women with severe chronic hypertension require a more intensive management program that includes medication.

We're sure you are wondering whether this medication will be safe for your baby. This is an important question to ask. If you took blood pressure medication before you got pregnant, your obstetrician might want to work with your regular doctor to change it to one that is known to be safe during pregnancy. It's essential that you take the medications you need during pregnancy—just be sure that your obstetrician knows what they are and approves them. Although they cross the placenta and enter the baby's circulation, they may be necessary to prevent conditions such as uncontrolled high blood pressure. Discuss all of your medication with your doctors and ask any questions you might have about their effect on your unborn baby.

GESTATIONAL HYPERTENSION

As we explained, gestational hypertension is high blood pressure that first occurs in the second half of pregnancy—after 20 weeks. Women with this condition usually do not experience symptoms such as headaches, visual disturbances, excessive amounts of protein in their urine—which is associated with preeclampsia—or the excess weight gain that occurs in preeclampsia. Women with gestational hypertension do, however, run a higher risk for developing preeclampsia (discussed later in this section). In fact, 50 percent of women diagnosed with gestational hypertension at the six- to nine-month mark develop preeclampsia.

TREATING GESTATIONAL HYPERTENSION

Doctors treat women with mild gestational hypertension by carefully evaluating and closely monitoring the conditions of mother and baby for the duration of the pregnancy, sometimes prescribing medication, though not always. If blood pressure elevates to a potentially dangerous level, a perinatologist is usually called in. The ultimate decision about whether to deliver the baby early depends on how far along the pregnancy is, the status of the unborn baby's health and the severity of the mother's condition at the time of evaluation.

Noelle's Gestational Hypertension

When Noelle, age 20, was 8 months pregnant and at a routine prenatal care visit, she had a blood pressure reading of 155/90. Her obstetrician had her lie on her side for ten minutes, hoping to see it drop to a safer level, but this had no impact. The second reading was 155/95. Noelle was suffering from gestational hypertension, though she was emphatic about feeling fine and exhibited no symptoms. She couldn't believe it—she'd always associated hypertension with her elder relatives who took "pressure pills," as she put it.

Noelle and her baby were in danger; even at her young age, the condition made Noelle susceptible to stroke or preeclampsia. Because she was about 32 weeks pregnant, her doctor prescribed bed rest and close observation. He was hesitant to prescribe medication unless her blood pressure rose above 155/100. Unfortunately, a week or so later, Noelle's blood pressure was 155/105, so she was put on medication. She also consulted a perinatologist, who observed her closely and monitored her baby's growth. While Noelle and her doctors managed her care, her baby's lungs had time to mature. Those few weeks were critical because at 36 weeks, Noelle's perinatologist determined that her baby wasn't growing anymore and advised her obstetrician that it was time to deliver.

Although baby Kyla didn't quite make it to 37 weeks inside her mom's womb, she emerged a fully viable, healthy baby, needing only a few days in the NICU before she could go home with Mom and Dad.

Preeclampsia

When hypertension develops at or after 20 weeks of pregnancy with symptoms that indicate that the mother's organs are being impaired, the condition is known as preeclampsia. The symptoms can include headaches, vision disturbance, swelling in the hands, feet and face, and rapid weight gain. The name of the disorder literally means "prior to eclampsia" (or seizure) because when blood pressure is high enough to damage organs, the patient is at risk for seizures.

Although it occurs in less than 10 percent of all pregnancies, preeclampsia is more common in black women and those pregnant for the first time. In fact, preeclampsia strikes earlier and more severely in black women. It is also more prevalent among mothers of multiples and those with chronic hypertension, diabetes or kidney disease. The causes of preeclampsia are still unknown.

Preeclampsia is considered severe when blood pressure is 160/90 or higher and accompanied by symptoms such as severe headaches, blurred vision, abdominal pain or epileptic seizures. This condition can be very serious. Left untreated, the mother is at risk for a stroke or even death due to uncontrollable bleeding, heart failure, kidney failure or fluid in the lungs as a result of swelling. However—and this is a big however—women who receive regular prenatal care *rarely* suffer from these devastating complications because obstetricians look for the warning signs at each visit. This is one of the many reasons why good prenatal care is so important.

TREATING PREECLAMPSIA

Managing preeclampsia is a great challenge. If you develop it in your ninth month, you will be hospitalized and possibly given a course of magnesium sulfate—to prevent seizures—both during and after delivery. If you develop it prior to your ninth month, you will probably still be hospitalized and cared for by an experienced obstetrician or perinatologist.

PREECLAMPSIA SUPERIMPOSED ON CHRONIC HYPERTENSION

This rather wordy disorder signifies that preeclampsia has developed on top of already diagnosed chronic hypertension. What you need to understand about this condition is that your health can decline quickly, and your doctors must make decisions about your treatment and overall care rather abruptly. If immediate delivery is seen as the best option, you might be scheduled for a cesarean section rather than risk the time it takes to induce your labor.

Babies born to mothers who have chronic hypertension with superimposed preeclampsia will more than likely need time in the NICU level three or level four because of early delivery. And although this prospect can be quite upsetting, we'd like you to think about this situation from a "glass half full" perspective. We are very fortunate that medical technology has evolved to the point where our vulnerable premature babies are safe in the NICU until they are ready to go home. It's reassuring to know that 80 percent of the babies delivered after only 28 weeks in the womb (about 7 months' gestation) do well. Please believe us when we tell you that most of the babies whose lives were saved by skilled neonatal teams—including doctors called neonatologists and neonatal nurses—go on to be healthy children with little to no lingering evidence of a shaky start to life. Yes, there is a lot to be grateful for even under these conditions.

Jamie's Preeclampsia Superimposed on Chronic Hypertension

Jamie was 31 when she became pregnant for the first time. She knew she had inconsistent high blood pressure prior to pregnancy but had never required medication to control it. During her fourth month of pregnancy, Jamie's blood pressure was elevated to the point where her doctor opted to put her on antihypertensive medication. When she asked him whether she could continue to work, he said yes but that she should try to take it easy.

Jamie's blood pressure continued to rise, so her doctor increased her medication and prescribed bed rest. Unfortunately, this course of action did little to control her ever-rising pressure, and she began to experience weight gain, headaches, swelling of her hands and feet, and an excessive amount of protein in her urine. Jamie was suffering from severe preeclampsia. Action had to be taken. At 7 months, baby Sasha was born by cesarean section weighing 2 pounds, 11 ounces. From her first days in the NICU, Sasha did well and is now a healthy, happy little girl. If you were to meet her, you would see no evidence whatsoever that she was born prematurely. Thanks to the effective emergency care Jaimie got, Sasha can now kick a soccer ball as far as any boy her age.

Asthma

"Oh no! I can't stop coughing, and I feel like I'm losing my breath. Is this part of the pregnancy, or am I having an asthma attack?"

Asthma symptoms are scary enough when you're *not* pregnant; add an unborn baby to the scenario and the thought of not being able to breathe becomes unbearable. Don't worry, though. Whether or not you are a chronic asthma sufferer, there are a lot of things you can do to control breathing problems and maintain your health and that of your unborn baby.

WHAT ASTHMA IS

Asthma is a chronic lung inflammation disorder that causes swelling and a narrowing of the tubes that carry air into and from your lungs. The resulting symptoms are shortness of breath, wheezing and coughing. The changes that occur within the lungs during an asthma attack make exhaling more difficult than inhaling—thus the familiar wheezing sound.

Asthma attacks may be triggered by an allergic reaction, cigarette smoke, infection, cold air, mold, cockroaches, dust mites, animal dander, exercise or even emotional stress.

HOW ASTHMA AFFECTS PREGNANCY

The connection between asthma and pregnancy isn't simple. Some pregnant women find their symptoms improve—though most experience the opposite. Naturally, oxygen levels are a major concern for unborn babies, so if you suffer from asthma, it's important to discuss this with your health-care provider.

Asthma sufferers are divided into four categories based on the frequency and severity of their symptoms:

1. Intermittent
2. Mild persistent
3. Moderate persistent
4. Severe persistent

This table from the ACOG provides more details:

Asthma Severity	Symptom Frequency	Nighttime Awakening	Interference With Normal Activity
Intermittent (well controlled)	2 days per week or less	Twice per month or less	None
Mild Persistent (not well controlled)	More than 2 days per week but not daily	More than twice per month	Minor limitations
Moderate Persistent (not well controlled)	Daily symptoms	More than once per week	Some limitations
Severe Persistent (very poorly controlled)	Throughout the day	Four times per week or more	Extremely limited

Studies indicate that complications during pregnancy from asthma are most likely to arise during the third trimester, at the time of labor or right after giving birth. But generally speaking, the more severe the condition is before pregnancy, the greater the likelihood of symptoms during pregnancy.

Complicating matters is the fact that shortness of breath and labored breathing are common symptoms of a normal pregnancy. It's easy to see how asthma might put a pregnant woman's respiratory system under increased strain. The key to coping with this problem is to work with your physician to keep it in check and avoid these potential consequences:

- Pregnancy-induced hypertension
- Preeclampsia
- Greater risk of C-section delivery
- Maternal illness or morbidity (death)

What's more, an unborn baby can suffer from the following complications:

- Intrauterine growth restriction: limitations to the unborn baby's normal growth potential while in the womb, which can lead to poor health or even death of the fetus
- Low birth weight
- Preterm birth

Clearly, a lot can go wrong when asthma isn't controlled during pregnancy, so let's discuss the steps you can take to avoid these nasty complications.

TREATING ASTHMA DURING PREGNANCY

Asthma in a pregnant woman is typically comanaged by her obstetrician, a perinatologist and sometimes a pulmonary specialist (skilled in diagnosing and treating disorders of the lungs). These physicians work together to make sure that both the patient and her unborn child maintain an adequate level of blood oxygen during gestation and delivery. Their objectives can be summarized as follows:

• To maximize the pregnant woman's lung function

• To eliminate or control the triggers that can cause symptoms or attacks

• To educate the patient so that she can take part in her own care

• To administer medication as needed, but in as low a dose as possible

Many women worry about the effects of asthma medication on their unborn babies, and those concerns are valid. But the National Asthma Education and Prevention Program has found that "it is safer for pregnant women with asthma to be treated with asthma medications than it is for them to have asthma symptoms." Clearly, the risks and benefits must be weighed carefully—and that calls for the advice of a professional.

Here's another thing to keep in mind: inhalants are the most frequently used asthma treatment option during pregnancy—and for good reason. They are effective at reducing swollen airway tubes and preventing asthma attacks while having little effect on an unborn baby.

In addition to prescribing inhalant medication, a pregnant woman's medical team will probably advise peak flow monitoring throughout her pregnancy. Peak flow monitoring is a way of measuring lung function with the help of a small portable device called a peak flow meter. The patient blows hard through a mouthpiece at one end and the force of the air expelled is measured in liters per minute.

Regular peak flow monitoring can signal the constriction of the airways even before asthma symptoms can be felt—which is extremely useful in preventing asthma attacks and minimizing symptoms. Medication can be adjusted and administered proactively, preventing attacks before they occur.

There are some additional steps a pregnant woman can take to manage her asthma:

• Avoid coming into contact with substances that can cause an attack, including pollen, dust, smoke, mold, some animals and cleaning products. (If you suffer from asthma, you are probably well aware of your own triggers. Stay away from them!)

• Identify the first signs of breathing difficulties and treat them promptly.

• Communicate regularly with your doctors so that your medication can be adjusted as you proceed through your pregnancy and delivery.

Gestational Diabetes

"There's sugar in my urine?"

Gestational diabetes sounds alarming, but it is one of the most common complications of pregnancy.

WHAT GESTATIONAL DIABETES IS

Diabetes is a disorder in which the person isn't producing enough of the naturally occurring hormone insulin to change sugar (or carbohydrates such as bread, potatoes, rice and pasta) into energy. As a result, too much sugar ends up in the bloodstream and urine. When a woman develops this disorder for the first time during pregnancy, it's called gestational diabetes.

Women who have diabetes prior to pregnancy can be type 1 diabetics, which means they acquired the disease during childhood, or type 2 diabetics, which means they acquired the disease during adulthood. If you have diabetes prior to pregnancy, it's very important that you consult with your physician about it early and often during your pregnancy. (It's definitely a must to talk over with your doctor if you are contemplating getting pregnant. It's never too early to prepare for a healthy pregnancy.) Whether you have diabetes going in or develop it when pregnant, it is critical to keep your blood sugar level in check during the first 2 months, otherwise it can cause serious abnormalities in your unborn baby.

If you do suffer from diabetes or are at risk of it due to your family history or other risk factors (see below), your glucose level—the amount of sugar in your urine—should be checked at your first prenatal visit and at every subsequent one until delivery. Even if you carry no risk factors for diabetes, all women are screened for the disorder at 24 to 28 weeks (7 months) using one of two tests: the one-hour 50-gram glucose challenge test (GCT) or the two-hour 75-gram GCT. If the results indicate any sign of the disorder, your doctor will then order a three-hour 100-gram glucose tolerance test (GTT). If these results are abnormal as well—don't panic—you probably have gestational diabetes.

The following situations will put you at risk for gestational diabetes:

- Being part of any nonwhite race
- Being obese with a BMI of 30 or more (see Chapter 2)
- Having had gestational diabetes in previous pregnancies
- Having previous unexplained stillbirths
- Having a family history of gestational diabetes

HOW DIABETES AFFECTS PREGNANCY

While it's true that gestational diabetes comes with the risk of certain complications, that doesn't mean you can't have a healthy baby—as long as you take care to manage the condition carefully with your health-care provider's help. The risks to your health and that of your baby are directly related to the sugar levels in your body. Left uncontrolled, they can cause preeclampsia or diabetes later in life, or necessitate a C-section delivery. Risks to your unborn baby include:

- **Macrosomia.** An unusually large baby due to excessive sugar passing through the placenta, which converts into excess fat and muscle and enlarged organs. Labor and delivery of a baby with macrosomia are quite difficult, and there is an increased risk of injury to the woman's birth canal. The baby may also suffer from a lack of oxygen or from nerve damage during delivery, resulting in neurological impairments or arm paralysis. Although babies with macrosomia are large, they tend to have immature lung function and difficulty breathing (respiratory distress syndrome). They can also be listless and limp, feed poorly and may suffer from the sudden withdrawal of sugar, a condition called hypoglycemia.
- **Shoulder dystocia.** This occurs when the baby's head is delivered vaginally but his or her front shoulder gets stuck behind the mother's pubic bone.
- **Respiratory distress syndrome.** Difficulty breathing at birth.
- **Neonatal hypoglycemia.** Low blood sugar levels in the newborn due to the sudden drop-off in the amount of sugar traveling to the baby from the mother in utero.

To reduce or even eliminate the risk of these complications, maintaining strict control over sugar (glucose) levels is critical right up until delivery.

Gestational diabetes usually disappears after delivery—but if you continue to have a problem metabolizing sugar and carbohydrates after pregnancy—or if the problem recurs years later—you are very likely a diabetic and will have to seek treatment for the condition. This has been known to happen in some women, but don't worry too much about it. You probably know a number of people with diabetes who are living full lives under the care of a specialist who can prescribe the proper medications and testing.

TREATING GESTATIONAL DIABETES DURING PREGNANCY

Early diagnosis of gestational diabetes is one of the first and most important steps in treating the disorder, followed by counseling and education about proper management of sugar levels. Understanding the condition and how to treat it is critical because most of the care you get as a pregnant woman is *self*-care, and you want to feel empowered to take the best possible care of yourself and your baby.

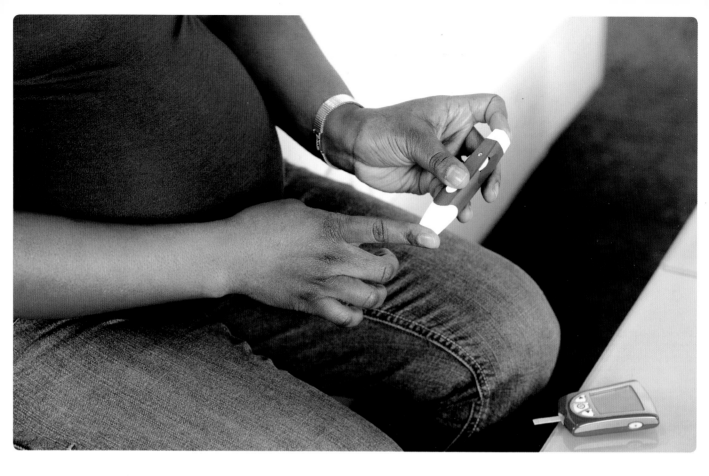

Gestational diabetes is controlled either with a special diet alone or in combination with medication. Diet recommendations are based on your BMI, but three meals plus one or two snacks per day is typical. Generally speaking, 33 to 40 percent of your diet should be carbohydrates, 40 percent should be fats and 20 percent should be proteins. It's also important that you eat on a regularly timed schedule. Because it can be tricky to figure out exactly what to eat under these conditions, it's a good idea to consult with a dietitian or nutritionist.

Continual monitoring of sugar levels is an important component of care for pregnant women with gestational diabetes. Many health-care practitioners suggest self-glucose monitoring at home at various times throughout the day. After all, the first step in controlling sugar levels is knowing what they are—and in a diabetic, they can swing widely in a short period of time.

If your physician finds that your condition cannot be controlled by diet alone, she or he may prescribe insulin as part of your treatment plan. There are a number of insulin therapies available; your health-care provider will determine which one is most appropriate for your individual needs.

Your doctor will also begin fetal surveillance at around 7 to 8½ months, administering such tests as the non-stress test (NST) or ultrasound. Checking on the baby's condition and development in this way can help ensure his or her ultimate health and well-being.

The NST involves monitoring the pattern of the unborn baby's heart rate and is usually performed weekly for women requiring insulin.

Estimation of the baby weight before delivery may be determined by physical exams or ultrasounds. This estimate becomes important for a fetus considered large (over 9 pounds) because a C-section may be required. A biophysical profile of the baby—determined by using an ultrasound to measure the amniotic fluid and check up on the baby's activity level—may be obtained also.

When gestational diabetes has been controlled throughout pregnancy by diet alone, fetal surveillance may not be necessary and the obstetrician may move forward with natural labor.

Coral's Diabetes

Coral was 34 when she became pregnant for the second time. She had experienced gestational diabetes during her first pregnancy, so it wasn't a surprise that the GTT she took at 7 months came back abnormal. She had gestational diabetes again.

Coral remained calm about it, knowing she'd had a good result the last time. She consulted carefully with a dietitian, and then religiously stuck to a diet she hoped would allow her to manage her diabetes without the use of medication. Coral's discipline and dedication paid off! Little Christian was born at term, vaginally, weighing a healthy 8 pounds, 6 ounces.

Preterm Birth

"No stroller, no crib; guess who's sleeping in a dresser drawer?"

Besides catching us unprepared, premature babies require a lot of medical attention. We're very fortunate that advances in medical care have upped the odds for babies that show up ahead of schedule.

WHAT PRETERM BIRTH IS

When babies are in the womb for less than the optimal 9 months, we say they are preterm or premature. This condition is further broken down into categories based on just how early they are. If a baby is born at 24 to 34 weeks, she or he is early preterm; a baby who arrives at 34 to 37 weeks is late preterm.

The ACOG discourages delivery of a baby before 39 weeks unless medically necessary, as preterm birth can be dangerous. Premature infants are often small and thin, their heads appearing too large for their bodies. There is little fat under their skin, making it difficult for them to maintain a normal body temperature and necessitating the use of an incubator. They may also suffer from respiratory distress if their lungs haven't developed fully. They often have poor sucking and swallowing reflexes, making intravenous (into the veins) feeding necessary. The premature baby's digestive tract may not function well either, which can lead to other complications.

Some causes of prematurity include a weak cervix (as described in the section on preterm labor), infection of the amniotic fluid, the presence of fibroids and substance abuse.

PREVENTING PRETERM BIRTH

Preventing preterm birth may involve preventing or stopping preterm labor, covered in the section above. But if there is no stopping your baby from coming early, stay calm and listen to your medical team. Nowadays, babies who come into the world sooner than expected are well cared for and most survive and thrive.

PRETERM LABOR

Preterm labor can be frightening, but you should know about some dramatic medical advances designed to prevent or stop it.

WHAT PRETERM LABOR IS

Preterm labor occurs when a pregnant woman is experiencing uterine contractions and her cervix dilates (opens) earlier than three weeks prior to her due date, allowing her baby to enter the birth canal. If she isn't treated, she may give birth prematurely (as discussed above in Preterm Birth). A number of factors increase a woman's chances of having preterm labor:

- A history of preterm birth
- A short cervix (prior to pregnancy, the cervix is closed and inflexible; it gradually softens and shortens as the mother progresses toward labor and birth.)
- A "weak cervix," one that cannot carry a pregnancy to term
- A pregnancy soon after childbirth
- Prior surgery on the uterus or cervix
- Being underweight or overweight
- Smoking or using drugs during pregnancy
- Multiple fetuses (twins, triplets, etc.)

It can be difficult to diagnose preterm labor, but if you carry one or more of the risk factors, watch for these symptoms:

- Increased vaginal discharge, either watery or bloody
- Lower-back pain
- Abdominal cramps
- Contractions
- A gush or trickle of fluid that might indicate your water has broken

Regularly timed contractions certainly seem like early labor, but it's important to understand the difference between Braxton-Hicks, or "false," contractions (see Chapter 12 for more on these) and the ones that indicate the onset of labor. If you think you might be in labor, contact your medical professional, who will probably want to check your cervix for softening and dilation—the primary indicators of impending labor. He or she may also test your vaginal secretions for the presence of a protein known as fetal fibronectin. This glue-like substance helps connect your unborn baby's amniotic sac to your uterine wall. It starts to break down naturally when you are preparing for delivery, so its presence may be an indication that you are going into labor.

TREATING PRETERM LABOR

If you are at high risk for preterm labor, your doctor may restrict your activity and prescribe abstinence from sexual intercourse, home contraction monitoring or medication. If you have a "short cervix," your doctor may even stitch your cervix closed to prevent it from opening prematurely under the pressure of your growing baby.

If you sense that you may be going into premature labor, call your doctor immediately, time your contractions, drink plenty of fluids and restrict your activity until further instructed. Your doctors may decide to:

- Administer antibiotics to treat infection of the amniotic fluid
- Use tocolytic drugs to stop your uterine contractions
- Prescribe medication to help speed up the maturation of your baby's lungs
- Give you magnesium sulfate to help reduce the risk of neurological impairments such as cerebral palsy that can occur in babies born too soon

Nichole's Preterm Labor

Nichole was 31 when she became pregnant for the third time. She had experienced preterm labor and delivery due to a weak cervix twice before. This time her doctor stitched her cervix closed when she was 4 months along and prescribed progesterone (a medication to strengthen the cervix). When Nichole complained of pain during her seventh month, her doctor instructed her to go to the hospital, where it was confirmed that she was experiencing preterm labor contractions. Naturally, this worried her, but Nichole went home with a positive attitude and obeyed her doctor's order of strict bed rest. Baby Ethan made it all worthwhile when he came into the world at 9 months, weighing a healthy 8 pounds, 3 ounces.

Preterm Premature Rupture of Membranes (PPROM)

"What is this? I know I couldn't have wet myself, but it's way too early for my water to break."

Just like preterm labor, premature rupture of membranes (PROM) can be a very scary development. If you find yourself in this situation, have faith in modern medicine and keep telling your little one to stay put.

WHAT PPROM IS

To understand this disorder, let's first start with the sequence of labor events. The first stage of labor and the second stage of labor occurs when a woman is fully dialated. Typically, at some point prior to the second stage of labor a woman's membranes rupture—her "water breaks." If this happens before she goes into labor, she is considered to be experiencing premature rupture of membranes, or PROM. When a woman's membranes rupture, she experiences either a sudden gush or continuous leakage of clear fluids from her vagina. But it isn't always crystal clear that this is due to ruptured membranes. If you find yourself unsure of whether your membranes have ruptured, it's best to notify your health-care practitioner immediately. A doctor can confirm suspicions of PROM by analyzing your history and administering various tests.

There are two kinds of PROM, depending on how far along a woman is in her pregnancy. If she has been pregnant for 37-plus weeks, but her water breaks before her labor starts, she is considered to have term PROM. If she has been pregnant for fewer than 37 weeks when her water breaks, she is considered to be experiencing preterm PROM (PPROM).

PPROM, may be linked to one or more of the following factors:

- Undetected uterine contractions
- History of PPROM in previous pregnancies
- Second- or third-trimester bleeding (see the definition of *third trimester bleeding* later in this section)
- Cigarette smoking
- Illicit drug use
- Low body mass index (see previous discussion in Chapter 2)
- Shortened cervical length
- Infection of the amniotic fluid
- Multiple births
- Fibroids (see later in this section)

When the barrier between the pregnant woman and her unborn baby is broken before labor, there is a higher chance that bacteria from the woman's cervix or vagina will travel upward to the baby's amniotic membranes and umbilical cord. Without the protection of a closed amniotic sac, the bacteria can cause serious infection or fever for mother and baby. Such infections are called chorioamnionitis (*KOR-ee-oh-AM-nee-oh-ni-tis*).

Women with chorioamnionitis usually have a fever during labor, foul-smelling discharge, uterine tenderness, elevated white blood cell count and fetuses usually have elevated heart rates. These dangerous infections cause neonatal deaths and long-term neurological problems in children.

TREATING PPROM

Women experiencing PPROM are usually admitted into the hospital for evaluation and careful monitoring. Health-care providers quickly seek to determine the age of the unborn baby, his or her position in the womb, the presence of fetal distress or infection, and the condition and viability of the placenta. In cases of term PROM, doctors proceed to deliver the baby in order to prevent infection. The same is usually true for women who are 34 weeks pregnant or more. Management of PPROM—when the woman is less than 34 weeks pregnant—often involves the use of electronic fetal monitors to observe and watch for abnormal fetal heart rate and uterine contractions. If the mother is anywhere from 24 weeks to 34 weeks along, doctors will administer antibiotics to prolong the pregnancy for as long as they feel is safe, monitoring her closely and doing all they can to prevent infections.

A pregnancy faced with PPROM at less than 23 weeks is extremely challenging for the unborn baby. Doctors essentially watch and wait for progress or proceed with delivery if they determine that is the safer option. Babies born this early can survive but often face a host of complications. Most seriously, their lungs tend to be underdeveloped, which can lead to respiratory distress, infection and brain hemorrhage.

Third-Trimester Bleeding and Postpartum Bleeding

"I'm bleeding!"

The sight of blood is probably one of the scariest things a pregnant woman can experience. But while it should certainly be taken seriously, it is usually manageable.

WHAT THIRD-TRIMESTER BLEEDING IS

The definitive source of bleeding during the last 3 months of pregnancy often remains a mystery, but there are three probable causes: placenta abruptio, placenta previa and placenta accreta.

PLACENTA ABRUPTIO

Placenta abruptio is the premature separation of the placenta from the uterus either before or during labor, often just before delivery. This is a life-threatening condition for mother and baby because of the extensive blood loss that occurs at the site of the separation. Although its exact cause is unknown, risk factors for placenta abruptio include preeclampsia, PPROM, high blood pressure, carrying two or more babies, cigarette smoking and cocaine use.

Bleeding from the site of the separation usually causes abdominal pain, tenderness and the onset of continuous contractions. A complete separation of the placenta from the uterine wall necessitates an emergency C-section to safeguard the life of the fetus. Partial separation may cause only moderate bleeding and may not jeopardize the baby's well-being as long as the flow of his or her oxygen to the placenta and passage of nutrients remain unaffected.

PLACENTA PREVIA

Placenta previa occurs when the placenta attaches to the uterus in an abnormal way—either near or covering the birth canal opening. This condition is usually identified early in the pregnancy with the help of an ultrasound and can cause some painless bleeding in the third trimester. The danger associated with placenta previa is that blood loss can become severe during dilation of the cervix, when the placenta may begin to separate from the uterine wall.

There are three types of previa: complete, partial and low-lying. Complete previa refers to a placenta that has grown completely over the birth canal opening. Partial, or marginal, previa refers to a placenta that partially covers the cervix opening. Low-lying previa refers to a placenta that has attached itself close to the cervical opening.

PLACENTA ACCRETA AND RELATED CONDITIONS

Placenta accreta occurs when the placenta has attached itself so deeply into the uterine wall that it doesn't separate spontaneously during the third stage of labor. In some cases, placenta increta occurs, which is when the placenta actually works itself all the way through the uterine wall. Very rarely, the placenta can work its way through and beyond the uterus, attaching itself to another organ such as the bladder. This is called placenta percreta.

As you can imagine, these conditions put the mother and baby at risk for serious blood loss during labor when it is time for the placenta to separate from the uterus. Some 90 percent of patients with these conditions require blood transfusions during labor and delivery.

TREATING THIRD-TRIMESTER BLEEDING

PLACENTA ABRUPTIO

Management of placenta abruptio depends on the gestational age of the unborn baby when it occurs and the amount of blood the mother is losing. If the bleeding is mild and the pregnancy close to term, the doctor may opt for vaginal delivery. If the bleeding occurs relatively early in the third trimester, the doctor may attempt to avoid premature delivery by restricting the mother's activity and observing her closely for signs of distress. If hemorrhaging and blood loss are severe, an immediate C-section is the best course of action regardless of the maturity of the baby.

Keep in mind that hemorrhaging at any time during a pregnancy is a sign that something isn't quite right. If you see red, call your health-care provider right away and be prepared to tell her or him how heavy it is and what other symptoms you are experiencing.

PLACENTA PREVIA

Management of placenta previa depends on the amount of blood loss, the location of the placenta and the gestational age of the baby.

If there is excessive bleeding, regardless of the baby's gestational age or the location of the placenta, a C-section is performed. If the placenta covers the cervix, a C-section will be scheduled for before labor begins to avoid the consequences of a dilating cervix.

If the placenta is low-lying, the patient may be allowed to go into labor and deliver vaginally, though she will be observed carefully in case a last-minute C-section may be required to preserve the health of mother and baby.

Placenta accreta, increta and percreta are considered high-risk conditions and don't offer a range of options. C-section delivery is necessary and is usually performed at 34 weeks in a medical center equipped to provide extensive transfusions if required. Any woman diagnosed with one of these disorders would be wise to discuss the situation in detail with her doctor prior to her scheduled C-section. The doctor may broach the possible necessity of removing the uterus—hysterectomy—during the surgery. As radical as this may sound, it is better to talk through the possibility ahead of time, rather than wake up to a devastating surprise.

Fibroids

"Just how much room do I have in there? I'm home to fibroids and a growing baby, too!"

Fibroids really seem to have their way with us black women in particular. The good news is that in most cases they are quite benign. The bad news is that during pregnancy, they can compete for space with the baby as he or she develops.

WHAT FIBROIDS ARE

Uterine fibroids are generally noncancerous tumors, balls of fibers and connective tissues that typically grow on the inner uterine wall. They can also grow on the outer surface of the uterus or within the wall itself. Fibroids can grow larger than a grapefruit or remain as small as a pea, and (alas) they are quite resilient, thanks to their own rich blood supply.

The hormone estrogen helps fibroids thrive, which is why they usually shrink after menopause, when estrogen levels drop. African American women are three times more likely to develop fibroids than white women, and often at an earlier age. No one knows what causes fibroids or why they are particularly rampant among African American women, although heredity may play a role. If you have them, chances are some of your female forebears did, too.

Many women experience no problems due to their fibroids, but some women report long and painful periods, fatigue due to anemia, constipation, pain during intercourse or frequent trips to the bathroom caused by pressure on the bladder. And, most serious of all, fibroids can cause infertility by blocking the fallopian tubes or preventing the fertilized egg from implanting itself in the uterine wall or lining. They may also cause miscarriage if they are large and positioned within the lining of the uterus.

Elaine's Fibroids

Elaine knew she had fibroids and discussed them with her doctor when she became pregnant with her third child at age 30. She was also aware of the attendant risk of preterm labor. She took it easy throughout most of her pregnancy, knowing there was little she could do other than remain vigilant for any symptoms.

During her eighth month, she started feeling pain in her abdominal area. After speaking with her doctor, she went to the hospital. Sure enough—she was having contractions. She was treated with intravenous (IV) fluids, allowed to rest and told to limit her activities until the baby was full term. Elaine followed orders and gave birth vaginally at term to a healthy baby boy weighing 7 pounds, 5 ounces.

HOW FIBROIDS AFFECT PREGNANCY

Fibroids affect unborn babies directly when they are large and located so as to make it hard for the baby to move into the head-down position prior to birth. These babies end up in positions that often require delivery by C-section.

Depending on the size of the fibroids and where they are, they can also cause the placenta to attach in an abnormal location within the uterus during the first few weeks of pregnancy. This condition is called placenta previa. In placenta previa, the placenta partially or completely covers the birth canal—a challenging condition for both baby and mother that necessitates a C-section. Detachment of the placenta as the cervix widens during labor can cause a dangerous loss of blood. Fibroids can also cause extreme pain and preterm labor and birth.

TREATING FIBROIDS DURING PREGNANCY

If a woman with fibroids is experiencing no pain or complications that might affect the baby, her physician will probably do nothing but monitor the situation. If she is experiencing severe pain, she may have to restrict her activity and take pain-relief medication.

In rare cases, minimally invasive surgery may be performed at the time of delivery to remove the fibroids—but only if the doctor believes they would compromise a successful delivery. This type of surgery is called a myomectomy. For obvious reasons, it is better if a woman has a myomectomy before getting pregnant to avoid the potential risks outlined above. If a woman has had myomectomies prior to her pregnancy, she may be scheduled for a C-section between her 37th and 38th week of pregnancy to reduce the risk of rupturing those old surgical scars due to the stress of labor and delivery.

Low Birth Weight

"My baby is so tiny!"

Your body possesses a brilliant process for developing a perfect human being. Sometimes we weaken that process by creating conditions that are avoidable. Not all complications are avoidable, but some are. And in most cases low birth weight is one of them.

WHAT LOW BIRTH WEIGHT IS

Babies born weighing less than 5 pounds, 8 ounces are considered low birth weight (LBW) babies. They may have been born prematurely or their intrauterine growth (in-womb growth) may have been delayed or restricted. According to the National Center for Health Statistics, the rate of LBW babies among African American newborns is slightly less than double that of white babies and of most other racial groups.

Babies who weigh less than 3 pounds at birth are at risk for birth defects, physical and mental disabilities and respiratory problems. In addition, very LBW babies may also develop behavioral, learning, visual and hearing problems later on in life.

As you know, it's the nutrients and oxygen from the mother's blood that nourishes and supports her unborn baby. If blood flow to the placenta is abnormal, lacking in either nutrients or oxygen, the baby's development will probably be impaired. Weakened maternal health and inadequate nutrition are the usual culprits that can jeopardize a woman's ability to support her unborn baby.

What weakens maternal health and nutrition? In far too many cases it's a compromised quality of a pregnant woman's life. Ongoing hardship and life struggles constantly chip away at good health. Low pre-pregnancy weight, insufficient weight gain during pregnancy, cigarette smoking, substance abuse and the lack of proper prenatal care will put a precious baby at risk for low birth weight, so it's vitally important for Mom to take care of herself before, during and after pregnancy.

THE UNDERWEIGHT WOMAN

As we discussed in Chapter 2, your weight directly affects your overall health. Once you've determined your BMI by using the method we've described, you will know whether you are underweight, overweight or within healthy norms. If your BMI is 18.5 or less, you are considered underweight—and that can be as threatening to a pregnancy as being overweight.

There is no set amount of weight that an underweight woman should gain during pregnancy. If you're underweight, you'll have to consult with your health-care provider to figure out what's best for you. And it isn't just a matter of eating more; it's about eating right. Your doctor will undoubtedly offer recommendations about your diet or might suggest that you consult a nutritionist to make sure you are gaining weight in a healthy way to lessen the risk of having a baby with LBW. A common recommendation is to add 20 grams of protein and 500 calories to the usual nutritional requirements of a pregnant woman.

INSUFFICIENT WEIGHT GAIN

You know that weight gain during pregnancy is normal and inevitable—but how much is the right amount when attempting to avoid the risk of giving birth to a baby with LBW? It cannot be stressed enough: your unborn baby needs the proper "building blocks"—nutrients and oxygen—in order to grow, and they all come from you. Without a healthy and sufficient diet, you cannot produce a healthy baby. And of course that involves gaining some extra weight beyond the weight of your developing fetus.

The nausea and vomiting that are common in the early months can make it hard to gain weight at first. That is perfectly normal. But a woman who has gained fewer than 10 pounds by her fifth month is often considered to be putting her baby at risk. If you are concerned that you might not be putting on enough weight, talk to your doctor about it. She or he may have a specific meal plan to recommend or may send you to a nutritionist to get one.

CIGARETTE SMOKING

We all know that cigarette smoking is bad for us in any circumstance—but did you know that it can cause preterm births and babies with LBW? This is one of the most avoidable risks discussed in this book. We can't say it strongly enough (and the mandatory warning on every cigarette pack confirms it): smoking cigarettes while pregnant has a devastating effect on the unborn baby.

Babies born to women who smoke during pregnancy are small—often at or below the tenth percentile in weight. That means that 90 percent of other babies weigh more! Babies of smokers are twice as likely to be born with LBW as those of nonsmokers. Why? Because the carbon monoxide the mother inhales when smoking decreases the amount of oxygen delivered to the placenta, your baby's life support. Additionally, nicotine tightens the arteries of the smoker, reducing blood flow. And that affects the flow of life-giving nutrients to the baby.

And the problems don't end with childbirth. When a smoker nurses her baby, she is delivering nicotine through her breast milk—to say nothing of the secondhand smoke the baby is inhaling by living under the same roof with a smoker. For that reason, it is best if others in the household refrain from smoking as well.

We know it's tough to quit. You may have tried and failed in the past, but it is more important now than ever, so try again. Talk to your doctor about some of the quitting aides and methods currently available and find out what might be safe to try during pregnancy. And if you simply can't give up smoking altogether, you have to shoot for sharply reducing the number of cigarettes you smoke each day. Two very important lives are depending on it!

COCAINE ABUSE

No judgment here, just harsh reality. Cocaine and crack readily cross the placenta and are major health risks to both mother and unborn child. In addition to increasing the risk of having a baby with LBW, using cocaine during pregnancy can cause spontaneous abortion, preterm delivery, PPROM or PROM, or placenta abruptio. Statistics show that 25 percent of substance abusers deliver prematurely and 22 percent of babies born to drug users exhibit LBW. Beyond that, the effects on the baby can be devastating, including heart, urinary and genital defects, intestinal problems, strokes and poor feeding. All of these are a result of the fact that cocaine constricts a pregnant woman's arteries, thereby reducing blood flow below adequate levels.

And there are risks for the mother, too, including heart attacks, strokes, seizures, malnutrition, hepatitis and sexually transmitted diseases. It may not be easy, but we urge you to be honest with your health-care practitioner about any dangerous habits or addictions you may suffer from. Like us, your doctor is not there to judge you but will want to help you get a handle on things for your own sake and that of your baby.

INADEQUATE PRENATAL CARE

Poor prenatal care can put your baby at risk of LBW, so keep those appointments with your health-care provider and heed his or her advice all the way. The kind of careful monitoring of your baby's development that we have described throughout this book is very important, as are the prescriptions and preventive measures your doctor may recommend. Without the help of a trusted professional, you and your baby may be vulnerable to a wide variety of diseases and disorders that can be managed or avoided altogether.

Get the picture? You are too valuable a person to have compromised health, and your baby is too precious to have to pay for it if you do. Yes, life struggles are no joke and for some of us they can seem too hard to manage without a bad habit. But you are an intelligent woman and one who just might be growing the next president of the United States. Eat well, sleep soundly, relax and start to get a grip on those habits—as difficult as it might be. It will all be worthwhile, we promise.

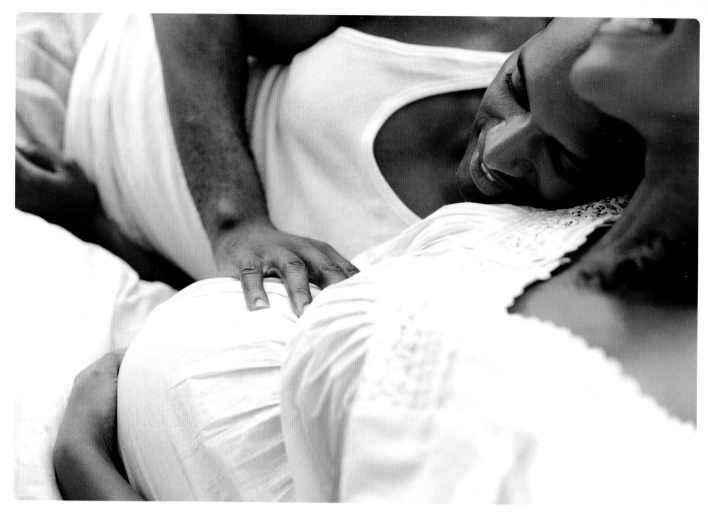

CHAPTER 4

You Are Still a Beautiful Sexual Being with Needs & So Is He!

All through your first trimester, you may be thinking, "I'm nauseous, I keep vomiting and I'm tired. Ain't nothing going on but the rent." This is the reality for many women, and it's normal. Most couples report a decrease in sexual activity during the first trimester, primarily because of the physical discomforts of early pregnancy. Come your second trimester, though, things may be looking up in that department. Your breasts aren't so sore anymore and the increase in your vaginal secretions, brought on by your hormones, can heighten sexual arousal. "Bring it!"

But—as you know—sex is more than a physical experience. Your desire for sex and your ability to perform sexually are affected by a variety of things. So even if you and your partner are both feeling fine physically, there may be some emotional or psychological issues interfering with your sex life during pregnancy. Maybe you look in the mirror at your swelling midsection and just don't feel attractive. Your man may have some issues about the way you look, too, though he is probably smart enough to keep that to himself!

On the flip side, there are some psychological benefits of pregnancy sex, too. There's certainly no fear of getting pregnant; that issue is off the table, along with the need to deal with birth control devices or medication. And if you were trying to get pregnant, that stress is behind you as well. You and your honey can enjoy a sense of sexual freedom now, perhaps for the first time in your lives.

Some couples are afraid that sex may hurt the baby, and that can be a turnoff by anybody's standards. We encourage you to talk this over with your health-care provider, but the bottom line is this: sexual intercourse during an uncomplicated pregnancy should not be harmful to you *or* your unborn baby in any way. You should know by this point if your pregnancy is likely to be a complicated pregnancy because your doctor has taken your full history, examined you thoroughly and discussed your health status with you—and will continue to do so at each prenatal visit.

So where does this leave you when it comes to having healthy, satisfying sex during pregnancy? It comes down to understanding some basic facts and communicating with your partner. Know what to expect, talk about it with your man, and as long as your decisions are informed ones, you can safely and freely do what feels good for both of you.

Here's what to expect physically. As we said, most women do experience a decrease in sexual desire in their first trimester for obvious reasons. No one feels sexy or aroused when throwing up or totally exhausted. The last three months of pregnancy can bring a decrease in desire as well. Fatigue returns because of the excess weight you're carrying around, you may be experiencing back pain or heartburn, and there's a whole lot of movement going on inside your much larger midsection. Sometimes it's difficult just finding a comfortable position to sit or lie down in, let alone have sex in! So by process of elimination, your second trimester will probably be when most of the action takes place.

But we urge you not to ignore each other's physical needs during the first and third trimesters of pregnancy. (That's six whole months total, after all!) You may not be feeling very sexual, but you can still be very sensual. Intercourse doesn't have to be the objective of every encounter; instead, try focusing on the cuddles and caresses you both need. Body massages and long soaks in a warm bath can be great runners-up to sex. Communicate your desires to your man and suggest alternatives rather than expect him to know what you need on his own, especially if these activities were not how the two of you expressed your love before your pregnancy.

Not sure how to begin? Here are a few tips on massage, which can do wonders for the pregnant woman and the expectant father as well. The following techniques are being described with the pregnant women receiving the massage from her mate. In all likelihood, she too can perform them on her man. Receiving is always wonderful, but giving pleasure is magical as well.

The Power of Touch

Massage is a form of structured touch that communicates caring while easing the aches and pains of the pregnant body. Unfortunately, in our society we tend to underestimate the power of touch, probably because it becomes confused with sex. A sensual home massage between you and your mate forces you to create the time and the space to be together. It isn't goal-centered like sex, which many see as a means to achieving orgasms. Massage can be a fulfilling substitute for sex when you aren't feeling strictly sexual—or a valuable addition to it when you are. (And if your massage session turns into something more sexual, go for it—as long as it is mutually agreeable.)

Set the stage for a sensual massage session by appealing to your other senses. Eliminate interruptions—and that means phones *all the way* off. (We all know how annoying the sound of a vibrating cell phone can be.) Dim the lights. Warm the room. Select some background music that's soothing to both of you.

Next, select an oil or lotion that pleases you. Oil enhances the massage by allowing the masseuse's hands to glide effortlessly over the contours of the body. We suggest that you choose from the wide array of scented oils available, as these unleash the power of aromatherapy. A pleasing scent can actually change or create a mood. But if oil doesn't do it for you, talcum powder can be used instead.

Begin by lying close to each other, perhaps in a spoon position with your man on the outside. Synchronize your breathing and enjoy just being together for a little while as you relax and focus on the here and now of *you*.

Once you are both relaxed, your man can begin stroking and kneading your body in a variety of ways. Here are some ideas to get you started:

- Lie on your side with a pillow supporting your head and neck and one between your knees to support your upper leg. Your mate then places his hands side by side at the nape of your neck and glides them downward using long soothing strokes along the sides of your spine, fanning hands out at the lower back and gliding them back up. This should be repeated at least three times—more if you are enjoying it.
- Using both hands, your honey makes wide circular curves over your body.
- The soothing "cat stroke" involves slowly stroking down the body with one hand following the other, barely applying pressure so that the hands barely touch the skin.
- Kneading movements (think about kneading dough) can stretch and relax tense muscles, improve circulation and help eliminate waste—all of which you probably need as a pregnant woman. Kneading is most beneficial to the shoulders and the fleshy areas of the hips and thighs.
- Kneading is similar to wringing out a towel; you gently grasp the flesh, then push and pull it at the same time. The legs, thighs, lower back and buttocks are additional ideal locations for kneading a pregnant woman.
- Massage can be a godsend if you are experiencing backache. This type of massage is usually performed as you lie on your stomach. Obviously, that won't be comfortable or even possible during the later months of your pregnancy, so try lying on your side with cushions under your head and upper leg. Another option is to straddle a chair and lean your upper body and head against a pillow. (Make sure the back of the chair is high enough to support you.)

One last note about massage: make sure to avoid massages to your stomach area and don't engage in any massage if you have experienced bleeding or preterm contractions. If your pregnancy is high risk or if you have a pre-existing condition such as high blood pressure, you should speak to your health-care provider before indulging.

Relax, enjoy—and improvise! If it feels good, it probably is.

Surprising Changes

During pregnancy, the amount of blood flowing to the breasts and vaginal area increases, which can make for more intense orgasms or even a first orgasm for some women. That's a beautiful thing that might make all those weeks of nausea worth it!

Don't be surprised to find colostrum, or "first milk," escaping from your nipples when you have an orgasm in the later months of pregnancy. The extra blood flow of the moment (on top of your increased circulation in general) causes your breasts to become engorged, and they may leak a little. It's perfectly normal and has no ill effect other than perhaps to freak the two of you out!

Vaginal secretions also increase throughout pregnancy, and that can come into play when you're sexually stimulated. Again, no real consequence to anyone. After all, who doesn't enjoy a bit of extra lubrication? But you may want to warn your honey about it, especially if he enjoys providing oral sex.

Making More Love

If you want lovemaking to be a part of your routine regardless of how big you are and how different it may feel, the following positions may help you experience optimum stimulation while compensating for your big belly:

- **The Spoons.** This position will help you avoid putting pressure on your abdomen and breasts, besides being super affectionate as it allows your partner to cuddle up behind you and stroke and caress you. It's also ideal because you don't have to be all that active to derive plenty of pleasure.
- **The Swing Around.** This is another one that helps you compensate for your growing belly. Lie on your back and swing your legs around your partner. He can enter you rather easily and still have his hands free for additional stimulation.
- **The Straddle.** Sitting astride your partner, either facing him or away from him, is a great way to avoid bearing his weight on your delicate body. In fact, any woman-on-top position allows you to control the speed of your lovemaking and depth of your partner's penetration, which can be particularly appealing during pregnancy.

During your orgasms, your uterus may experience contractions—and this can slow down fetal activity. Afterward, you may notice that your baby is more active than usual. No harm done here, as long as yours is a normal pregnancy with no complications.

When complications do exist, such as premature labor or contractions, premature rupture of your membranes or a history of preterm delivery, your doctor may suggest or insist that you refrain from sexual activity. Even early in your pregnancy, if you've been spotting, your doctor may invoke a no-sex edict. And if you are carrying more than one fetus, sex may be ill-advised (and hard to pull off!) during later months. And here's an additional word of caution from us: even in an uncomplicated pregnancy, absolutely never allow your partner to blow air into your vagina. While this may seem harmless, it can actually cause an air embolism—a pocket of air lodged or trapped in a blood vessel that blocks the flow of blood. These have been known to be fatal.

All of that said, don't panic about sex, just be sensible about it—and don't be shy about asking your health-care provider questions on the topic—or any topic at all, for that matter.

The special closeness you enjoy with your man doesn't have to be compromised because you're pregnant. For 9 months, your pregnancy is a part of your identity, including your sexual identity. As long as you have the okay from your doctor, you shouldn't let the baby hinder you from expressing your sexuality and sensuality. It may feel a little different, it may involve some new practices or positions, but it's still the two of you engaging in some very important bonding at a momentous time in your lives. So celebrate one another and the miraculous life you've created with your sexuality!

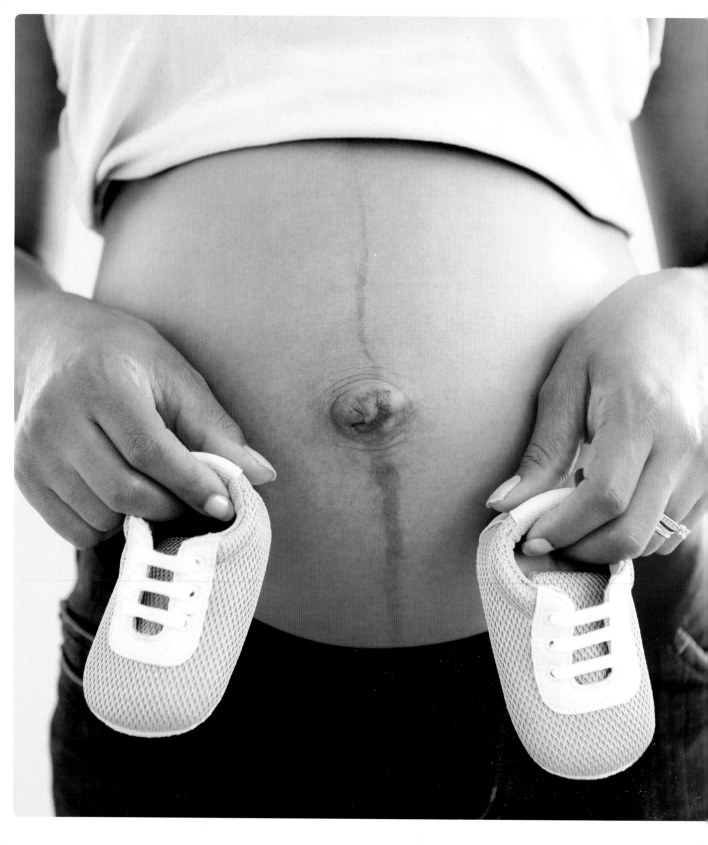

PART II

Your Pregnancy Month by Month

Every month of pregnancy is filled with dramatic changes and excitement. Here we'll provide a month-by-month explanation of some of the changes that you and your baby will experience. We hope it helps you celebrate this precious time in your life. We want to relieve some of your concerns about how your body feels and help you understand your baby's development. With that understanding, you can establish a relationship with your baby long before you hold him or her in your arms.

We've included some of the standard prenatal care routines as well as some new ones that health-care providers are using to ensure that women have a healthy pregnancy and a safe childbirth. So in addition to checking your blood pressure and weight gain during your monthly prenatal visits, your provider will be on the lookout for indicators that are known to seriously complicate childbirth. This is extremely important because although more mothers are surviving childbirth in developing countries, that is not the case here in the United States. Our survival rate is diminishing in the United States. That makes the Prenatal Appointment Schedule Worksheet in Appendix B more important than ever. It's an easy way to jot down answers to your questions and record those precious pregnancy milestones from each prenatal appointment with your provider.

Never to be taken lightly are those issues surrounding your pregnancy and your man, which is why we've included some key concepts to keep in mind regarding your relationship as you both proceed along your journey to parenthood.

It's been said that Africans were very much concerned with their deceased ancestors. Maybe it's because they realized just how much wisdom is taken with them when elders pass on. The "Wisdom from Our Ancestors" sidebars provide you with tidbits of information about what our great-grandmothers and great-great-grandmothers thought would sustain their lives and the lives of their unborn children during pregnancy and childbirth. It's entertaining and may also provide you with additional insight into the process of pregnancy and birth. The parallels between modern medicine and the practices of our ancestors are quite fascinating. Although some of their methods make sense and correlate to current procedures, some do not. This section is not about advice; it's about expanding your understanding of where we came from and being proud of what took place to get us here.

CHAPTER 5

The First Month
Weeks 1-4

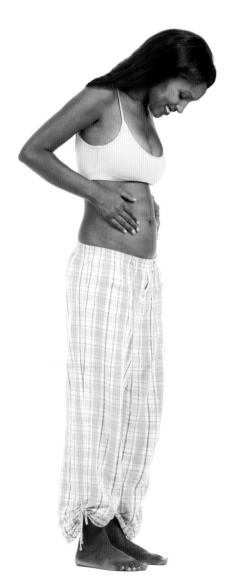

In these first weeks, you might have just discovered that you are pregnant. Congratulations! A flood of emotions may come over you now, even if it doesn't seem real to you yet. Your first few questions will probably be, *How far along am I?* and *When will my baby be born?* You may also start thinking about all of those baby names you always liked if you had a baby boy or girl of your own. And if he wasn't with you when you took those five home pregnancy tests (just to make sure), you will probably start to think about how you are going to break the news to the love of your life.

Once you have conceived, your ovulation and menstrual cycles will stop as a result of the pregnancy hormone human chorionic gonadotropin (HCG). HCG is a hormone that is released after the fertilized egg attaches to the uterine wall. Your body knows there's no need to ovulate since you are already pregnant, and you can't get "more pregnant." The hormone progesterone (*proJES-teh-rone*) is essential in helping your body adjust to pregnancy. It also causes the mucus between your uterus and vagina to become very dense and thick and develop into a plug. This very important mucus plug will help maintain the protective, enclosed environment that your baby needs in order to grow. It should remain intact until the beginning of labor.

How You Look

At one month you won't look pregnant, although your breasts may already be getting fuller and heavier than usual. (If you are an A-cup lady, you may absolutely love this.) You can expect your breast weight to increase by about 12 ounces during pregnancy—and the change is important as your body prepares to be able to feed your baby when she arrives. (Don't worry about the pronouns. We'll be switching genders from month to month.)

To protect your breast tissue from stretching and sagging, invest in well-fitting support bras regardless of how firm your breasts are now. And if your breasts are very large or have a tendency to sag, which can be genetic (thanks, Mom), you may also want to wear a lightweight bra to bed at night.

How You May Feel

Many women are not even sure they are pregnant at one month, but even this early you might be experiencing some physical symptoms like fatigue and nausea. You might also experience uncharacteristic mood swings and irritability. Is it PMS or is there a baby on the way? If you haven't yet confirmed that you're pregnant but have reason to suspect that you might be, it's time to find out!

Morning Sickness

"I just can't keep anything down."

Unlike its name suggests, the nausea and vomiting we call morning sickness aren't limited to just mornings. They can occur in the morning, evening or all day long. In fact, the phenomenon is a bit of a mystery: no one knows for sure what causes morning sickness or why it is worse for some women than it is for others. One theory suggests that it's caused by high levels of certain hormones, but others indicate that it might be due to changes in metabolism, emotional factors or fatigue. Whatever its cause, there is some agreement on how to deal with its symptoms:

- Have small but frequent meals.
- Even if you don't feel like eating, try to avoid having an empty stomach, since stomach acids will have nothing to digest but your stomach lining.
- Try eating crackers or toast before rising in the morning and turning in at night. This should also help regulate your blood sugar level, which is very important. If your blood sugar drops too low, you may become hypoglycemic, which can cause dizziness, weakness and blurred vision.
- If you can, try to keep your meals dry but alternate them with plenty of fluids in between. Some women find that eating and drinking at the same time puts too much strain on the digestive tract.

- Avoid the sight, smell and taste of foods that make you feel nauseous.
- Try a higher-carbohydrate diet, including such foods as whole-grain breads, brown rice, dried beans and peas.
- Get extra sleep and relaxation to avoid emotional drain and fatigue.

If nausea and vomiting become excessive and you experience signs of dehydration such as dry mouth and a strong smell to your urine, contact your practitioner. You may be in need of medical treatment.

Fatigue

"There's nothing like that pregnancy sleep."

You're likely to feel bone tired during the first few weeks of pregnancy, and this exhaustion may continue throughout the first trimester. Is it any wonder? Your body is working harder than it ever has, developing your baby's life-support system; the placenta. Once you've adjusted to the dynamic physical and emotional demands of pregnancy—and after the complete development of the placenta (by the second trimester)—you'll probably find you have more energy.

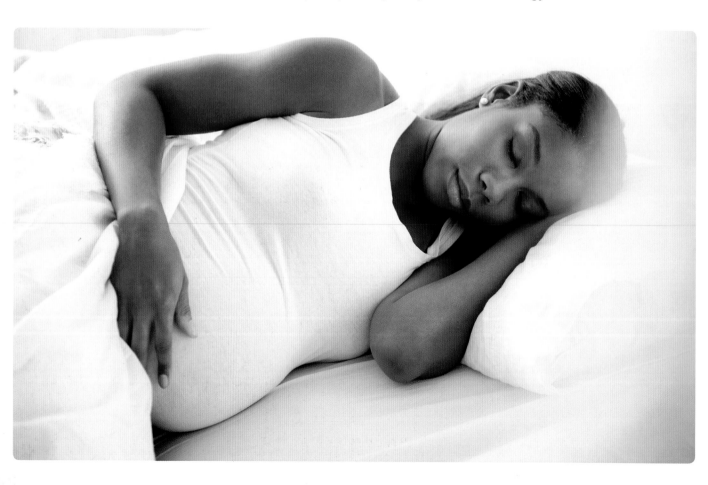

During this early phase, it's important to listen to your body and give it as much sleep as you can by turning in early and taking naps. And be sure to feed yourself well, too. Avoid foods with "empty calories" and no real health benefits, such as candy, caffeine and cake. You may find yourself craving these things for the temporary energy boost they offer, but once this "kick" wears off, your blood sugar level will drop, and you'll feel worse than before.

Get some exercise. If you're not the type for quick naps, a brisk walk or exercise routine can perk you up by improving your circulation. If you aren't sure what exercises are safe and beneficial during this time, there are a number of pregnancy exercise DVDs available. You might even find them at your local library. Many gyms and fitness centers offer exercise classes designed specifically for pregnant woman, so do a little research on that option as well, especially if you already belong to a club.

We have to add a disclaimer here, though you probably know what we're going to say. Never begin any type of exercise routine without first speaking about it with your health-care provider. There are a number of conditions that can arise during pregnancy that might make exercise dangerous for you or your baby, so get the official OK first!

Frequent Urinating

"You have to go again?"

You will probably hear this a lot from those closest to you. These frequent trips to the bathroom are caused by the pressure of your growing uterus on your bladder. It's a bother, for sure, but it won't last forever. Once your uterus rises into your abdominal area during the second trimester, your poor bladder won't be under so much pressure. The bad news is that this relief is temporary as well. As you reach your third trimester, the frequent urge to urinate will probably return.

To maintain good urinary health, go to the bathroom whenever you feel the urge, no matter how frequently it may be. You may want to increase your fluid intake during the day and decrease it in the evening to reduce the number of times your full bladder wakes you during the night, but make sure you are getting enough fluids overall, as they are important to your baby's health as well as your own.

Tender Breasts

"If I could just take them off and soak them."

Yes, a good soak in Epsom salt probably sounds pretty good right now. If your breasts are particularly achy, swollen and tender to touch, blame your hormones. The good news is that the soreness will fade away in a few weeks—certainly by your second trimester. Since there are no known cures for breast tenderness, you'll just have to avoid big bear hugs. You should also explain to your honey the need for a hands-off approach during lovemaking. Check your bra fit and comfort. You may need to invest in a better-fitting bra or even in an all-cotton sports-type bra for sleeping in at night.

Bloating

"OMG, I'm just a few weeks pregnant and I can't fit into my jeans?"

That may be true, but it's not the baby; it's gas. Your hormones are at it again. Progesterone relaxes the smooth muscles along your intestines, causing waste to stay longer inside of you, which can cause bloating and gas. Make sure you drink plenty of water, because being well hydrated aids digestion and helps prevent constipation. Avoid gassy foods such as cabbage and beans, and try having several smaller meals throughout the day rather than three large ones. That way, your digestive system won't get overloaded; it will have time to break down and process the food properly.

Strong Reaction to Odors

"Oh, that smell is killing me!"

Don't be surprised to find yourself reacting much more strongly than usual to certain odors. Pregnant women are known to have a heightened sense of smell. Common odors from foods or perfumes, even those you normally like, may now make you nauseous. It might be a whiff of meat on the grill, certain cooked vegetables, your dog or even your favorite hand cream. This new aversion is perfectly normal. There are some theories that explain why pregnant women are more sensitive to odors, although the evidence is limited and inconclusive. It is believed that your hormones strengthen the connection in your brain between your sense of smell and your emotional state. There is even some speculation that a heightened sense of smell is your body's way of protecting you from ingesting or breathing in substances that could be dangerous to the unborn baby. It is described as an evolutionary advantage. Regardless of why it happens, if it smells bad to you, try to avoid it. If you can't avoid it so easily, be prepared by sprinkling a few drops of a scent you do like on a tissue or handkerchief and keep it nearby. When your coworker's perfume is way over the top for you, try to cut off the nausea trigger with a whiff of your own more tolerable scent.

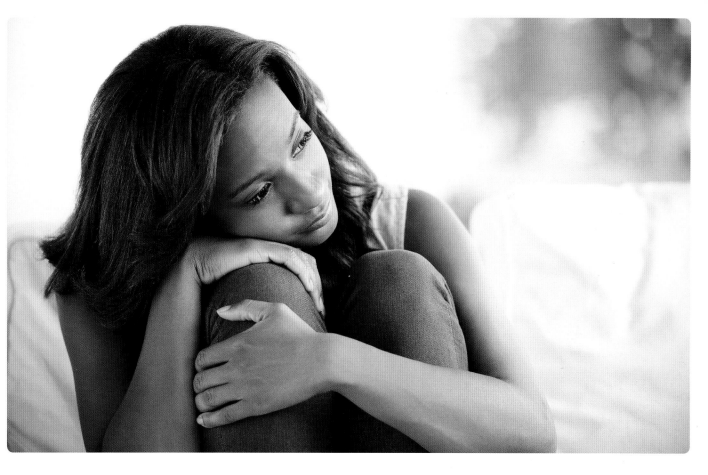

Ambivalence

"Will I be a good mom? Am I ready?"

Some ambivalence or uncertainty regarding your pregnancy is quite normal. You may experience all kinds of mixed feelings, including joy, regret, fear and elation—sometimes all in one day! These mood swings are quite common, especially during your first trimester, and pose no threat to you or your unborn baby. Although there is no cure for mood swings, you should avoid sugar and caffeine, since these can intensify such feelings (and we've already talked about their effect on blood sugar and energy swings).

No pregnancy is without the occasional twinge of anxiety over everything from stretch marks to the pain of labor. And there are those ever-present concerns about the financial realities of parenthood, too. Is there enough room in your house or apartment for a baby and all of the equipment that comes along with her? Cramped quarters can significantly up the anxiety level during pregnancy—but you know you'll work it out somehow.

Work has also been shown to affect a woman's feelings during pregnancy. If you are your family's sole means of financial support, the idea of taking time off and then having to juggle child care can be a daunting prospect. Just remember, as that new life takes shape inside you, you are not alone. There are many of us who have to take care of business for our families. Talk to some working moms you know, make sure you understand the maternity policies at your workplace (more about this in Chapter 1), and rest assured that millions of women all over the world manage to find a balance between being a mom and being a breadwinner. There are more resources for working moms in Appendix C at the back of this book.

It may sound like a generalization, but you know it's true: as African American women, we have a history of surviving and persevering in less than ideal situations. We all have well-worn stories about making a dollar out of fifteen cents at some point in our lives. This long-standing necessity to cope has its plus side in that we have developed inner strength that can come in handy during pregnancy and child rearing. But there are times when even the strongest black woman loses her ability to love and trust herself. That's when danger arises. If you reach the point where you don't feel you can cope with your life, you should seek help—for the sake of your baby as well as yourself.

Depression during pregnancy and right after giving birth affects one out of seven women. You are not alone. Depression is common and treatable, and far too many black women suffer from it. Talk to your health-care provider, or contact any of the organizations we list below. Your mind and spirit are precious during pregnancy—don't neglect them any more than you'd neglect your body.

If you have a pre-existing depressive disorder and take medication to control your symptoms, you may be tempted to stop taking it for fear of its effect on your unborn baby. Please don't do that without consulting your mental and physical health professionals. You, your therapist and your prenatal health-care provider must carefully weigh your options together to come up with the right solution. In some cases, a change in medication—rather than going cold turkey—might be the best bet for you and your baby.

If you don't currently have a psychotherapist but feel you might need one, there is no better time than right now to connect with one. Here are just a few of the agencies that focus on mental health for African Americans:

- The Association of Black Psychologists: www.abpsi.org
- Black Mental Health Alliance: www.blackmentalhealth.com
- National Organization for People of Color Against Suicide: www.nopcas.org
- Black Psychiatrists of America: www.bpaincpsych.org
- National Association of Black Social Workers: www.nabsw.org

If clinical therapy doesn't feel like the right move for you right now, you might want to try talking to a trusted member of your clergy or a supportive family member or friend. You can never have too much support from loved ones and trusted friends, so share what is on your mind.

Your Baby at One Month

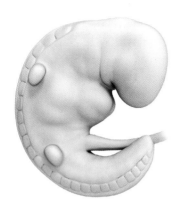

One week after conception, the fertilized egg is called a blastocyst (*BLAS-teh-sist*), which is really just a ball of dividing cells on its way to becoming your baby. As the cells multiply, they begin to play specific roles, some becoming part of the placenta and some the actual embryo. The blastocyst floats freely within the uterus for a few days after conception, and then it settles securely into your uterine lining. At this point, your body sends out messages to the rest of your body's systems. One of the most important ones goes directly to your immune system, which must adjust to the blastocyst and protect rather than reject it.

Once the blastocyst has attached itself safely to the uterus, and your body understands that it is there, the important work of developing your baby's life-support organs can begin. The changes that are occurring at this point are dramatic and critical to your baby's future development.

During the third week of life, the embryo, which is what your baby is now called, must divide into three layers. Each layer is responsible for the development of certain organs. The outer layer, or ectoderm (*EK-teh-durm*), is responsible for the formation of the brain, nerves, skin, hair and tooth enamel. The middle layer, or mesoderm (*MEH-zeh-durm*), develops into bones, muscles, heart, blood and blood vessels, kidneys and some reproductive organs. The inner layer, or endoderm (*EN-deh-durm*), forms the stomach, liver, intestines, lungs and urinary tract.

The fourth week after conception marks the beginning of another important period. It is during this time that your baby's heart chambers begin to fuse and beat for the first time. Your baby is now flexed in a *C* shape. One of the folds will become the head, and the other the bottom, which is shaped like a pointed tail right now. Between the two folds, the neural tube (site of the spinal cord) is growing, as well as the spine bones that will protect the cord. The nerve cells developing now will continue to grow even after birth until they span every inch of your baby's body. They are among the first cells to have a specific task, which is to coordinate the functions of all the other systems of the body.

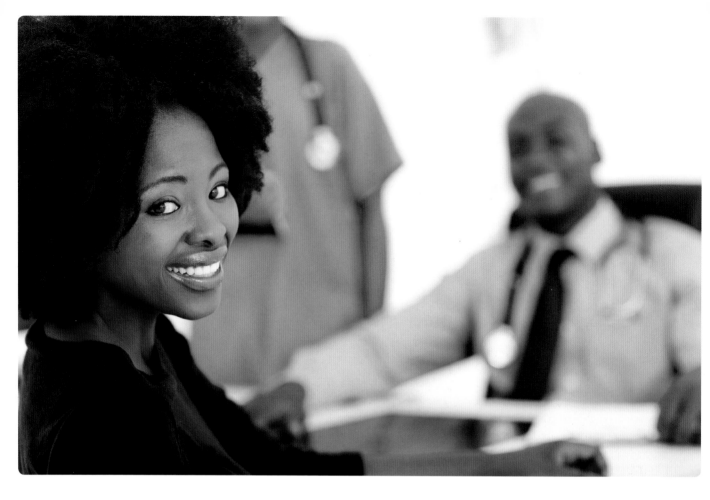

Your First Prenatal Care Visit

As you now understand, the first four weeks of your baby's life are very important to her survival. Although she'll need her full 9 months in your womb to develop fully and safely, one of the most important stages is the development of her heart and nervous system, and that is happening right now. Ironically, this is usually the time when we think least about our unborn baby, if at all, since many women may not even be aware that they are pregnant yet. If you know you are, even if you don't feel it yet, it's extremely important that you begin prenatal care.

Your first prenatal visit with your doctor, midwife or other practitioner will be the most comprehensive. After that, you will most likely be asked to visit once a month until your 28th week of pregnancy, and then every two weeks until week 36, when you'll be asked to visit once a week until you deliver.

You should schedule your first prenatal visit once you've missed your menstrual period and you suspect you're pregnant. Be prepared to cover a lot of ground at this first visit. Your practitioner will confirm your pregnancy, estimate your due date, identify any risk factors you may have, develop a plan for your prenatal care and delivery and establish a personal and professional relationship with you.

Confirming Pregnancy

Your practitioner can confirm your pregnancy with a blood or urine test, or an internal examination.

A blood test can detect pregnancy with virtually 100 percent accuracy as early as one week after conception by identifying and measuring the presence of hCG in the blood. This test can also help date the pregnancy. Be prepared to wait a few hours for your test results as, in most cases, your sample will have to be sent to a laboratory for analysis.

An in-office urine test is similar to the home pregnancy test you may already have taken. It can detect the presence of hCG as early as seven to nine days after conception with close to 100 percent accuracy.

The internal examination is a manual way to check for pregnancy. Your practitioner is looking for a softening of the cervix and enlargement of the uterus, both indicators of a baby on board. The nonpregnant uterus is flat, whereas the uterus of a woman who is 7 weeks into pregnancy is shaped like a hen's egg.

Your Estimated Date of Delivery

"When will my baby be born?"

The customary way to estimate a baby's birthday is by taking the first day of Mom's last menstrual period (LMP), subtracting three months, and adding one week and one year. So, if your LMP was December 1, 2015, your estimated date of delivery would be September 8, 2016.

Once an approximate due date is established, your health-care provider can monitor your baby's rate of development to be sure all is progressing normally. Equally important, you'll be able to plan your maternity leave and get all of your ducks in a row at home. But don't count on the little one arriving exactly on schedule. In addition to the fact that the date is just an estimate, babies can come early or late. There is some consensus in the medical field that it's best for an infant to reach between 39 and 42 weeks in the womb—but shorter terms can produce healthy babies, especially with the help of today's neonatal technologies, as discussed in Chapter 3.

Your Health History

During your initial visit, your practitioner will take a detailed history of your own health, including these elements:

- Your menstrual history, including the first day of your last period, regularity of your cycle and recent use of hormonal contraception.

- Your medical history, including any surgical procedures you've had; any problems with anesthesia, blood transfusions, allergies, medications; any medical disorders or psychiatric disorders. This is the time to discuss in detail how you'll manage any ongoing medical disorders such as anemia, high blood pressure, fibroids or asthma. If you and your doctor determine that you fall into the high-risk category, you'll decide together whether you should see a perinatologist.

- Your family history, including details about the presence of twins, hypertension, diabetes or genetic disorders.

- Your social history, including your marital status, living arrangements, family structure, financial status, health insurance and pregnancy concerns.

- Your obstetric history, including any factors that may influence your current pregnancy. Your doctor will want to know how many times you've been pregnant along with a detailed account of each outcome. Did you experience complications? Did you carry your babies to term? How big were they when they arrived? Answers to all of these questions and more will help your doctor know what to watch for this time around.

- Your contraceptive history, including what method you customarily use, whether your pregnancy was planned and how long it took you to conceive (if you were actively trying). This might also include a discussion about tubal ligation (tube tying) after you give birth, if you don't intend to have more children. Your consent is needed well in advance for this procedure, and a lot of thought (and consultation with your partner) should go into the decision. If you think it is something you might be interested in, it isn't too early to start talking about it.

The Physical Exam and Tests

This first prenatal visit should also include a complete physical examination. Your height and weight will be taken and used as a baseline against which to compare your physical changes over the next 9 months. Your caregiver will also want to examine your breasts and nipples and note the size of your pelvis, uterus and abdomen. Prenatal screening tests may also be administered based on the recommendations of the American College of Obstetricians and Gynecologists, as follows:

ROUTINE TESTS IN PREGNANCY

The tests recommended for all women during the course of pregnancy are designed to reveal any potential problems that might come up. Most of these conditions can be treated, and most of the tests are performed on samples of your blood and urine.

Blood tests can determine the following:

- Your blood type, which can be A, B, AB or O.
- Your Rh factor, which can be Rh-positive (most people are) or Rh-negative. The Rh factor is a protein found in red blood cells. This information is very important during pregnancy because problems can arise when a mother and her unborn baby have different Rh factors. Although you and your unborn baby have your own distinct blood systems, a small amount of blood does cross the placenta from baby to mother. When this happens, in the small percentage of women who are Rh-negative but carrying a baby who is Rh-positive, the mother will begin to make antibodies that fight the baby's Rh factor and may break down the baby's red blood cells. It sounds like a frightening situation—and it is certainly a serious matter—but it is rare that these antibodies end up causing serious problems for the baby. It is more likely to have an effect during a second pregnancy with an Rh-positive fetus, possibly causing anemia in the unborn baby, but by then, you and your doctor should be prepared to deal with any potential Rh factor complication.
- Whether you have anemia (a condition marked by a deficiency of red blood cells or hemoglobin in the blood).
- Whether you have rubella (also called German measles), based on signs of a past infection. This virus is most dangerous if a pregnant woman catches it during the first 20 weeks of pregnancy. It can cause miscarriage, stillbirth or birth defects such as hearing loss, brain damage, heart defects or cataracts. Luckily, rubella is a rare condition since we all should have been vaccinated for it during our school days.
- Whether you have hepatitis B virus, which can cause an infection that affects the liver.
- Whether you have syphilis, which is a sexually transmitted disease (STD) caused by bacteria. A pregnant woman can get infected with an STD just as a nonpregnant woman can become infected. Passing syphilis to an unborn baby can lead to serious health problems such as premature birth, stillbirth and in some cases death shortly after birth.
- Whether you have HIV, which is the virus that causes AIDS.
- Your glucose level, which is the amount of sugar in your blood—a determining factor for diabetes.
- Whether you are a carrier of cystic fibrosis, which is a genetic disorder that can be passed from parent to child.
- Whether you have diabetes, which is determined by administering an A1C test.

- Whether your unborn baby may develop a genetic disorder passed on by you or the baby's father. Genetic disorder screenings can determine whether your baby is at risk for the following:
  - Sickle-cell anemia, a genetic anomaly that makes red blood cells sickle-shaped, rigid and sticky. This makes it hard for the cells to do their job and carry adequate amounts of oxygen throughout the body.
  - Thalassemia, another blood disorder that creates an abnormal form of protein in the red blood cells responsible for supplying the body with oxygen.
    - Both sickle-cell anemia and thalassemia disproportionately affect black people in the United States. If a pregnant woman has a history of either disease, her prenatal care should be comanaged by a hematologist (a doctor who specializes in diagnosing and treating diseases of the blood) and a maternal fetal specialist.
  - Cystic fibrosis, which damages the lungs and digestive system.
  - Tay-Sachs, a rare disease that destroys nerve cells.
  - Fragile X syndrome, a genetic condition that causes intellectual disabilities and behavioral challenges in children.
  - Hemophilia, a disorder that prevents the blood from clotting efficiently.
  - Spinal muscular atrophy (SMA), a disorder that affects control over the body's movement caused by an insufficiency of nerve cells, called motor neurons, in the spinal cord.
- Your blood count. A complete blood count during pregnancy provides your doctor with valuable information about the kind and number of cells in your red blood (the cells that carry oxygen to the body's tissues and remove carbon dioxide and other wastes), white blood (the cells that protect the body against infection) and platelets (the tiny cells that help the blood to clot, especially at the site of a wound). Your red blood count will tell the physician whether you suffer from anemia, which can hamper your blood's ability to supply your body with sufficient amounts of oxygen.
- Urine tests can determine the following:
  - The level of sugar in your urine. The presence of sugar in your urine is normal during pregnancy, but a high level could be a sign of diabetes.
  - The amount of protein in your urine. If this is high, it might be a sign of a urinary tract infection or kidney disease. In the later stages of pregnancy, protein in your urine could be a sign of preeclampsia (a condition we discuss in detail in Chapter 3).
  - Whether you have ketones in your urine, which may indicate that your body is burning fat rather than glucose (a simple sugar that gives the body energy) for energy, because it isn't producing enough insulin (a hormone made by the pancreas that allows your body to use sugar for energy). This condition can be the result of uncontrolled diabetes.

This may sound like a lot of testing—but the good news is that most of the problems these tests are designed to detect are not serious if discovered and dealt with in a timely way.

To help you keep track of the important information that gets discussed during your prenatal visits, we've included a Prenatal Appointment Schedule Worksheet in Appendix B. Make a copy of the form every month and use it to jot down the questions you want to ask your health-care provider during any of your upcoming appointments. Be prepared to write down answers and some of your personal data that gets collected, such as your weight, blood pressure and test results.

Your Pregnancy & Your Man

Let's take a minute or two to focus on that beautiful, masculine man who helped create the human being growing inside of you. Although you clearly have the physical responsibility for your baby right now, he is expecting as well. That's right; he is as pregnant as you are, at least in an emotional sense. He'll be dealing with a lot of changes, too, and they may be causing him some anxiety.

In general, whenever there is consideration of what is, there is concern over what will be. Men tend to worry that a baby will interfere with what's good between the two of you—and during some phases of your pregnancy, that might be true. In the early months, you might feel sick and not your usual self. (We've talked about this already—it will pass.) Later, as your body blossoms, your desire for sex—and even your ability to engage in your favorite activities—may be hampered. It's important to keep your partner's very real concerns in mind and try to help him understand that you are still *you*, the woman who loves him, and you are doing all that you can to make him a priority. With good communication, you two can get through the physical changes together and face your future as a family with joy and optimism.

Remember those mood swings we talked about? Think about how those may affect your man. If he's used to having an even-tempered woman around, it may be a challenge to "go with the flow." And watching you get nauseous and throw up a couple of times a day may make him queasy as well. He may have to step up his emotional game a little, and he'll need your help to do it. Talk to him about your feelings, and tell him what you need. If it's space, so be it. If it's a foot rub, even better—you'll be touching. It's important to make him understand that if you are happy and relaxed, the baby will be better off—and isn't that what you both want?

Beyond his own happiness, your man is probably just as concerned as you are about the health of the baby—but he's somewhat removed from the process. You must make an effort to keep him in the loop about all that you are feeling and finding out about the baby's development. How will he know that his baby is doing well unless you tell him so? Welcome his concern and attention, even if it means tolerating fifteen calls a day to ask how you feel and if you've eaten. And conversely, if he seems distant or unconcerned, make an effort to involve him. It will pay off for all of you once the baby is born and you are the tight-knit family you were meant to be.

Try to be realistic about your partner's journey toward parenthood. The moment that pregnancy test came up positive, he was thrown into a foreign world. We're not saying he didn't want to bring life into this world with you, just that he has no reference for it. As girls, we have thought about motherhood and practiced playing mommy since we were kids. For many of us, nurturing comes easily. This is not so for most men. And some of our men, in particular, don't have memories of their own fathers to guide them. So, while you may have a lot of needs right now (and this book is mainly about addressing those), remember that he has needs, too.

Wisdom from Our Ancestors

Our great-great-grandmothers were amazingly astute about what the laboring woman needs to bring life into this world. We are the proof of that. But medical advances in obstetrics and gynecology have reduced morbidity and mortality rates for woman and infants exponentially. Babies are surviving—and that's a good thing! As pregnant women, we live in fortunate times, but it is instructive to look back as well.

In this recurring feature, we offer you a bit of folk history and some entertainment—and in some cases, endeavor to separate the myths from reality. So, enjoy some of the "old wives' tales" from our rich culture—but always consult your health-care provider before engaging in any kind of homespun test, remedy or intervention—whether you found out about it here or anywhere else.

A FLASHBACK IN TIME

How did our great-great-grandmothers manage to produce a strong black race without the benefits of modern medicine? When you look at the way they lived, you have to wonder. Think about this the next time you are feeling crampy or cranky or just plain mad about what's happening to your body.

Back in the day, pregnancy was not an excuse for any changes in a woman's life or activities. Very little thought was put into when a baby was conceived or when he or she was due or what could go wrong along the way. Some women made the connection between the stoppage of menstruation and pregnancy—but in cultures where little clothing was worn, the first sign of pregnancy was probably that growing belly, along with swelling of the veins (which also became hot to the touch), the appearance of Montgomery's glands (the tiny bumps around the nipples) and changes in the coloring of the face.

Before there were home pregnancy tests or doctor-administered blood tests, ladies had to figure it out on their own. And you know what? They did.

To Do This Month

A Quick Checklist

- ☐ Confirm your pregnancy with a trip to your health-care provider.

- ☐ Make a copy of the Prenatal Appointment Schedule Worksheet (page 210) and jot down your questions.

- ☐ Invest in a well-fitted support bra, if needed.

- ☐ Talk with someone if you are feeling depressed.

- ☐ Talk with your man about his feelings and yours.

— CHAPTER 6 —

The Second Month

Weeks 5-8

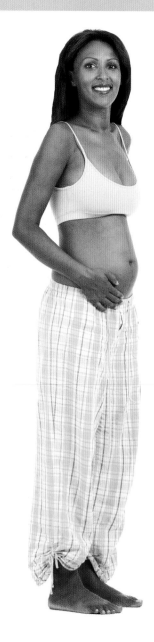

One of the purposes of this book is to help you understand and anticipate all of the extraordinary changes your body will undergo throughout your pregnancy—and of course they've already begun. But during the early months, these changes are more apparent to you than to others. In fact, if you've decided to wait a little while before making your big announcement to the world, it's unlikely that anyone will even know.

How You Look

That doesn't mean you aren't already feeling the changes. For starters, due to the extra hormones your body is producing, your skin may be going a little crazy. If you normally suffer from dry skin, it may be drier; if your skin is naturally oily, it may be even oilier. For that reason, you'll want to be sure that your skin-care products address your particular tendencies and help keep you glowing. Just be sure to read the labels on products carefully. You want to stick to products that are hypoallergenic and have been clinically tested to guard against skin irritation.

Dr. Sumayah Jamal, a New York–based, board-certified dermatologist we consulted, says that the most common skin conditions she sees in pregnant women are acne, chloasma gravidarum (*klo-AZ-ma grav-eh-DARE-um*), stretch marks and rashes.

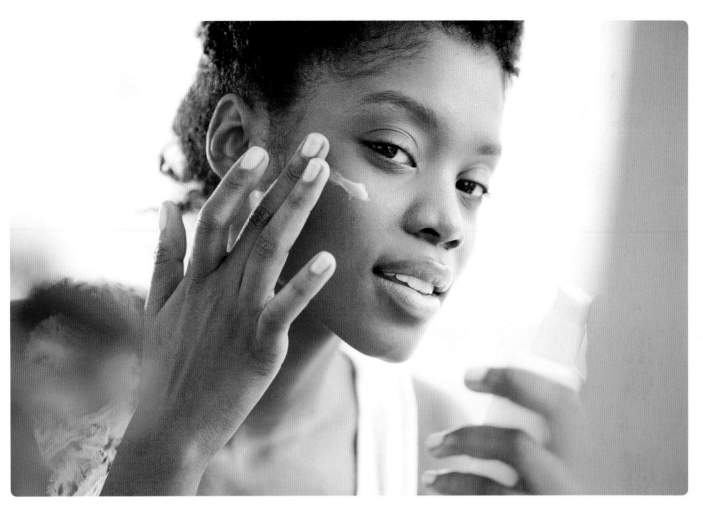

If acne is a problem for you, the good news is this: according to Dr. Jamal, noninvasive procedures such as facials and microdermabrasion (a nonchemical technique for removing dead skin cells) are perfectly safe during pregnancy. Acne can be caused by dead skin cells that clog the pores, so procedures and products designed to remove these skin cells can be very effective. Even chemical peels involving the use of glycolic acid and mandelic acid are safe during pregnancy, though they might sound a bit drastic. For those few women who develop large, inflamed cysts of the face, tiny drops of an anti-inflammatory can be injected to bring down the swelling and help with pain.

If you prefer a do-it-yourself approach to skin care, products such as facial cleansers, toners and moisturizers that contain glycolic acid can help control acne flare-ups. There are also a variety of topical prescription creams that are safe to use during pregnancy, including topical erythromycin and azelaic acid. If you prefer a more natural approach, Dr. Jamal recommends tea tree oil, available in any health food store, for help in ridding your complexion of pimples.

Why all of this attention to skin problems in a book on pregnancy? We have a reason. As Dr. Jamal stresses, acne tends to leave dark spots on black skin that can be long-lasting and difficult to treat. So, as a pregnant woman of color, it's a good idea to seek treatment from a dermatologist for serious acne flare-ups and avoid the possibility of permanent scarring. If you do find yourself with a dark spot, nonhydroquinone-based skin-lightening products such as kojic acid, licorice extract and azelaic acid can be used safely during pregnancy.

You can also cut down on those dreaded dark spots by avoiding the "pimple-pop-scar-makeup" cycle. We all do it. We get a pimple. We can't resist squeezing and popping it, and that leaves a scar or dark spot. We put on makeup to cover it, which in turn clogs our pores and causes another pimple—and the cycle starts all over again. Ladies, don't squeeze your pimples. If you promise to stop, we will, too!

We asked Dr. Jamal to recommend a particular skin-care regimen for pregnant women, and here's what she came up with: start with a fine exfoliating scrub to cleanse the skin, followed by a toner or—for more severe acne troubles—prescription cream. Use a good moisturizer and sunscreen during the day and a glycolic acid moisturizer at night. And again she recommends that all of the products you use regularly be hypoallergenic.

Chloasma gravidarum is a condition in which our bodies make too much beautiful brown pigment, and it shows up in patches on the face. This is not easy to treat during pregnancy, so if you are predisposed to it, it's best to minimize the effects by staying away from direct sunlight as much as possible—and we mean every part of you, not just your face. The sun tends to unleash those hormones that stimulate pigment production, so cover up and shade yourself, especially since the topical ointments often used to treat the condition are not recommended for use during pregnancy. And, for those times when avoiding exposure to the sun is impractical, Dr. Jamal recommends the following precautions:

- Apply sunscreen of SPF 50 or greater to all areas of the body that may be exposed to sunlight.
- Wear sunglasses. When sunlight hits the eye it can stimulate hyperpigmentation.
- Keep a wide-brimmed hat on your head; it can be one of your best protectors.
- Be aware of and avoid reflected sunlight as well. Even if you are indoors, sunrays pouring in through a window can create havoc on your face.
- Use a topical antioxidant serum such as vitamin C or E daily, along with azelaic acid, which slows down the production of excess pigmentation. (As we mentioned, you can also use safe skin lighteners such as kojic acid and licorice extracts.) Chemical peels that contain glycolic acid, lactic acid, phytic acid and mandelic acid are permissible as well.

Chloasma gravidarum is aggravating, for sure, but it's been known to clear up after the baby is born, and if it doesn't, you and your dermatologist have many more options for treatment once you no longer have precious cargo on board!

Let's move on to that mighty nemesis of pregnant ladies everywhere (and especially those of us of color): the stretch mark. We're sorry to report that Dr. Jamal hasn't found a miracle cream or oil that prevents this condition—and, honestly, nobody else has either, in spite of some of the claims out there.

There seems to be a genetic component to this skin disfigurement, so if your mom had stretch marks, you may be looking forward to them as well. Treatments, such as they are, will have to wait until after you give birth. At that point, laser treatments may improve the look of dark stretch marks as well as the lighter-colored ones, but it is extremely unlikely that the marks will go away completely.

Although most rashes during pregnancy are relatively harmless, some are more serious than others and can have an impact on the unborn baby. Dr. Jamal advises that any rash that develops during pregnancy should be evaluated immediately by a dermatologist.

How You May Feel

You may not have connected the dots because these conditions seem unrelated, but being pregnant can affect your breathing, blood circulation and vaginal discharge, even at this early stage in your pregnancy.

Breathing Difficulty

During your second month, you may experience difficulty breathing. This is because your lungs are in the process of adapting to be able to support your increased oxygen demands. Additionally, since your hormones are going a little crazy, you may have some swelling of the nose and throat, which can add to the problem. Although shortness of breath can be a little uncomfortable, this symptom isn't serious or long-lasting. You are a beautiful pregnant woman now, and that involves some annoying but benign changes in your health. Your best bet is to avoid over-the-counter drugs to alleviate this and other minor discomforts. (In other words, suck it up, sister!) But, of course, if the problem becomes intolerable, speak with your health-care provider about a safe remedy. Relief might be as simple as sleeping in a semi-sitting position propped up by pillows, or being more mindful of your basic posture as you sit at your desk.

Dizzy Spells

Your heart and blood circulatory system are going through some changes this month as well. Your total blood volume is increasing in direct correlation to your baby's weight and the development of his placenta. Your heart is beginning to work harder to provide adequate oxygen and nutrients to your baby.

Not all women get dizzy during pregnancy, but these changes to your circulatory system may cause dizzy spells. If the room starts to spin, move immediately to a seated position to avoid falling or passing out. By your second trimester, your body should adjust to these changes, and you'll have your legs under you again.

Increased Discharge

In early pregnancy, your cervix (the part of your uterus that connects to your vagina) and vagina soften and expel a watery discharge in greater volume than you are probably accustomed to. To relieve any discomfort, try the following:

- Wear cotton underwear, which breathe better and help keep you dry.
- Bathe regularly.
- Avoid douching, which can alter your pH balance.
- Avoid prolonged sitting, which can keep you damp.
- Use cornstarch to help stay dry.
- Avoid scratching if you begin to itch, so as to avoid irritation.

Your Baby at Two Months

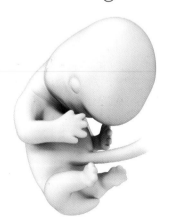

Eight weeks after conception, your baby has unquestionably human characteristics. During this month, his head is growing faster than any other part of his body, primarily because of the rapid development of his brain. His neck begins to develop, his tail disappears and his heart beats strongly at 140 to 150 beats per minute, approximately twice the rate of yours. His upper limbs also begin to develop identifiable hands, elbows and shoulders. His feet and toes begin growing, too, but they won't catch up to the functioning level of his arms and hands until well after birth. Your baby will be able to hold his bottle way before he can stand up and walk.

His eyes, eyelids and lenses are forming, and if you could look at him closely, you'd see additional indentations on his head where his nose and ears will develop. Believe it or not, by the end of this month—just the second month of your pregnancy—all of your baby's internal and external structures will be under construction, though still tiny and immature.

Prenatal Care at Two Months

At this month's visit with your health-care provider, he or she will probably check the following:

- Your weight
- Your blood pressure
- Your fundal height (the distance between your pubic bone and the highest point of your uterus)
- The fetal heartbeat
- Your urine for sugar and protein
- Your hands and feet for swelling, and your legs for varicose veins

Your provider may also perform a "dating ultrasound" this month. Your doctor will use the results to get a more accurate sense of how far along you are in your pregnancy and as a baseline for tracking your baby's growth and overall health over the next 7 months.

He or she will also want to know if you are experiencing any unusual symptoms and will address your concerns and questions—so, as always, come prepared!

One more thought: don't forget to take your folic acid. It's very important during the first 12 weeks of pregnancy in preventing birth defects of the spinal cord.

Your Pregnancy & Your Man

Most first-time fathers are delighted when they hear about a pregnancy. Many of them see it as an affirmation of their virility, or manhood, and you know that's a source of great pride for them. Your wonderfully virile man may also feel a sense of relief, presuming that the two of you were trying to conceive. The challenge of "trying to get pregnant" can be stressful, so if that's what you two were going through, it's time to celebrate. You knew you could do it—and you did!

But once you've clinked your glasses of ginger ale, buckle up and hold on, because pregnancy can send your emotions—his as well as yours—up and down faster than any roller coaster. At one moment your man may be beating his chest with pride over what good swimmers his "boys"

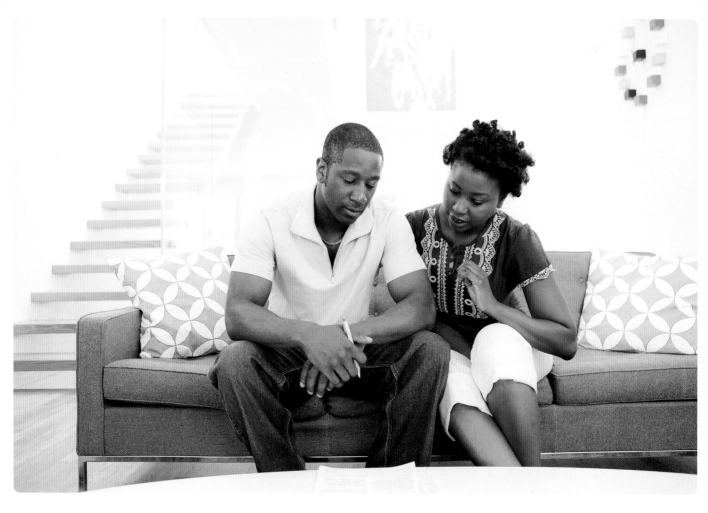

are, the next moment, he may be having these wildly irrational thoughts about whether the baby is even *his*. This concern is more common than you think, so put down the frying pan you were planning to use to knock some sense into him. His craziness probably has a lot to do with the fact that bringing life into this world is a huge responsibility, and at this point he has very little control over what's happening.

So how do you handle it? First, by keeping in mind that his real point isn't "I don't think that baby is mine;" it's probably more like, "I'm a little bit scared that I'm not ready to be a father." The best way to stay close is to share your honest feelings—so maybe your response could be, "Honey, sometimes I'm afraid that I won't know what I'm doing as a mother." The mutual experience of pregnancy and parenthood is a powerful one. It can bring you two closer together or drive you apart. If you want it to be that first thing, it's important that neither of you feels alone or abandoned with your feelings.

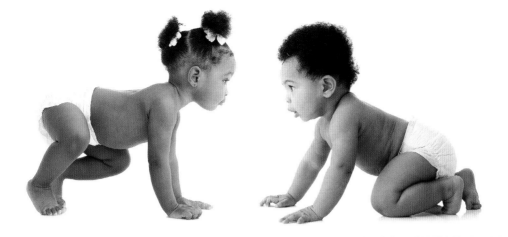

Wisdom from Our Ancestors
BLACK FOLK MYTHS & SUPERSTITIONS
IS IT A BOY OR IS IT A GIRL?

Predicting the sex of unborn babies is an age-old tradition that probably doesn't have much scientific validity but is definitely entertaining. Here are a few myths from our own ancestors about how to determine your baby's sex:

- If you carry the baby high and pointy, you're having a boy; low and round, it's a girl. (Or vice versa, depending on whose grandma you ask.)
  Reality Check: Just as a matter of fact, how you carry has more to do with your muscle tone and how your baby is positioned inside of you than anything else.
- If your pregnancy is obvious from the back, it'll be a boy, if not it's a girl.
- If the baby is lying toward your right side, it's a girl.
- Boys move around more in the womb.
- If you develop a little part in the back of your hair that won't go away, you're having a boy.
- If you feel good during your pregnancy, you're having a boy; if you suffer, it's a girl.
- If you feel unattractive, the baby is going to be a girl. Girls rob their mothers of their beauty, whereas boys do not.
- If a child dislikes you, then your baby will be the opposite sex from that child.
- If the baby is a girl, boys will give the pregnant woman much attention, whereas girls will practically ignore her.
- If your hair falls out during the time you're pregnant, the baby's going to be a girl. If your hair grows long and full, it will be a boy.
- If two children cling to you while you're pregnant, you'll have twins. If they're two girls, then you'll have two girls; two boys, then you'll have two boys; and the same if they happen to be a boy and a girl.

To Do This Month

A Quick Checklist

- ☐ Consult with a dermatologist for major acne flare-ups, if necessary.

- ☐ Start tolerating the minor discomforts of pregnancy.

- ☐ Make a copy of the Prenatal Appointment Schedule Worksheet (page 210) and jot down your questions.

- ☐ Go to this month's prenatal care appointment.

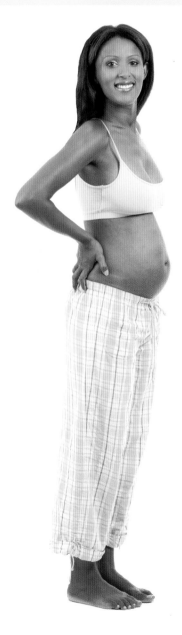

CHAPTER 7

The Third Month

Weeks 9-12

Well, your first trimester is almost over, and you're really beginning to feel pregnant. Many of the annoying discomforts that dragged you down the past couple of months are fading away now, and you can really begin to appreciate the beauty of this entire process. It's such a wonderful gift—enjoy it!

How You Look

Don't be alarmed if the tiny bumps around your nipples become larger and more visible this month. They're called Montgomery's glands, or sebaceous glands, and they're harmless. These glands actually produce an oily secretion to keep the nipple lubricated and protected.

You may also gain some weight this month, although probably not a lot. Due to the growth of your baby, the fundus, or base, of your uterus is beginning to rise above your pelvic bone. You can now feel your pregnancy by touching your stomach.

How You May Feel

You have extra blood flowing just about everywhere, which can cause you to experience some headaches now.

Numbness and Muscle Cramps

Increased blood flow is being distributed to your pelvic area, breasts and lungs. As a result, your legs, arms and brain may not be receiving the amount of oxygen they need for comfortable functioning. This can lead to numbness and cramping of the legs. If you experience these discomforts, try moving your legs vigorously or wearing support stockings. Some women even faint when they have been sitting or lying down for a long time and then get up suddenly. To prevent fainting spells, try to avoid sudden changes in your position; after prolonged sitting or lying down, try taking deep breaths as you rise slowly.

Bleeding Gums and Nose

Increased blood flow to your nose, throat area and lungs can cause nosebleeds, bleeding gums or a stuffy nose. How do you cope? Make sure your diet has adequate amounts of calcium and vitamin C. For bleeding gums, use a soft-bristle toothbrush and rinse your mouth with warm salt water a couple of times a day. You may also want to make an appointment with your dentist to remove the plaque on your teeth, as a way to promote gum health.

To help prevent nosebleeds, avoid blowing your nose vigorously. If you do experience a nosebleed, remain upright and pinch the nostrils together for 5 to 10 minutes. You may also want to keep your home nice and moist by using a humidifier or placing pans of water in your driest rooms.

Headaches

Some women experience headaches early in pregnancy. In most cases, no specific cause can be found. Higher blood pressure and hormone levels, eye strain, sinusitis and emotional factors may contribute. This form of discomfort is just one of many that we women must tolerate as society's bearers of life.

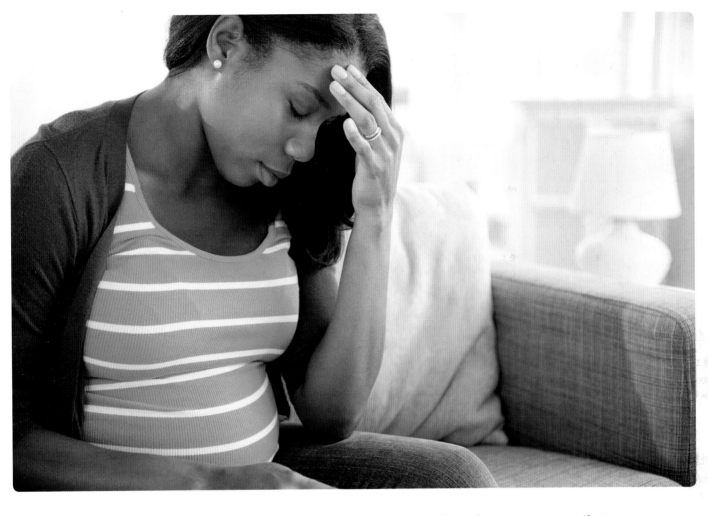

It is likely that your headache pain will go away as you proceed through your pregnancy. If you continue to have headaches, or if they are particularly severe, contact your caregiver. She or he may suggest that you take a pregnancy-safe pain reliever—but be aware that not all pain relievers are the same. Acetaminophen, the active ingredient in Tylenol, is routinely recommended during all stages of pregnancy. For short-term use, it's safe for you and your baby. It is always best to talk to your practitioner before taking any medication.

Your Baby at Three Months

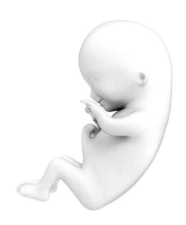

This month marks a significant milestone in your baby's development. All of the parts your little one will need for life have formed, and she is now called a fetus. You'll remember that last month was all about rapid head growth. Now body growth begins to accelerate.

At this point, the umbilical cord that joins you and your baby is fully developed. It has two arteries that carry waste and carbon dioxide from the baby to the placenta and one vein that carries nourishment and oxygen to the baby from the placenta. The placenta is connected to your body by the chorionic villi, tiny fingerlike projections that have attached themselves to the wall of your uterus.

During these early months, the fetus's blood supply comes from the yolk sac—a ball-shaped organ that makes blood for your baby until the marrow from her bones takes over that job.

Since the baby's intestines are too large for her abdomen at this point, they have formed outside of her body in the umbilical cord. Later on in your pregnancy, they will take their appropriate place in the baby's abdomen. This process is called an umbilical herniation and is a very normal part of development.

Your baby will start to form urine this month, which is released into the amniotic fluid. She may reabsorb some of this fluid by swallowing it (sounds yucky, but it's perfectly normal and harmless); the rest of it crosses the placental membrane into your own circulatory system.

Your baby may practice breathing now by inhaling and exhaling amniotic fluid. This respiration of fluid is instrumental in the proper formation of her lungs' air sacs. Your baby won't drown because she doesn't yet depend on her lungs for air. Her oxygen supply comes directly from you, through the placenta and umbilical cord. During this month, your baby's vocal cords complete their development—but without air from her lungs, she won't be able to cry aloud until birth.

Although her bones are growing and becoming stronger this month, your baby's ribs and backbone are still very soft and flexible. By the end of this month she will be able to kick her legs, make a fist, bend her wrist, turn her head, squint, frown, open her mouth and press her lips tightly together—all without you feeling a thing. It will take another month or so, when her bones are stronger still, before you will be able to feel her move.

Prenatal Care at Three Months

At this month's visit with your health-care provider, he or she will probably check the following:

- Your weight. At the end of your first trimester, the recommended average weight gain is about 4 to 5 pounds.
- Your blood pressure. It should be around 120/80 and not above 140/90.
- Your fundal height. This is usually measured with centimeter tape and the number of centimeters should be approximately equal to the number of weeks of gestation.
- The fetal heartbeat for strength and regularity.
- Your urine. Your health-care provider will be checking for sugar and protein.
- Any swelling of your hands and feet.
- Your uterine size and the growth of your fetus. Your caregiver will check these via manual palpation of the contours of your uterus.
- Prenatal screening tests. These may be suggested as early as month three if you have certain specific risk factors (see Chapter 8 for more on these).

Believe it or not, medical advancements have made it possible to screen unborn babies for possible developmental abnormalities as early as 10 weeks. Cell-free DNA testing, a sophisticated blood test that examines the unborn baby's DNA from its mother's bloodstream can recognize the indicators of a genetic disorder such as Down syndrome. The fact that it is noninvasive (as opposed to amniocentesis, which requires a needle inserted into your womb to remove a small sample of amniotic fluid) means that even pregnant women in high-risk categories can be screened for potential genetic disorders. Although amniocentesis is not a screening tool, it does offer accuracy in determining genetic disorders. The results of the DNA screening test can help a woman and her doctors determine if further testing, including amniocentesis, is advisable. Cell-free DNA testing is recommended for the following women:

- Women 35 years old or older
- Women whose ultrasounds indicate a possible developmental abnormality
- Women whose prior pregnancies have involved a genetic disorder
- Women with a family history of genetic disorder

It is important for you to understand that just because your doctor suggests that you take a DNA test or undergo amniocentesis, it doesn't mean that something is wrong. It also doesn't mean you have to comply; it is only a suggestion, albeit an expert one. As long as your decisions are informed—meaning that you have a good understanding of your situation, your options and the possible consequences—then they are likely to be the right ones for you and your family.

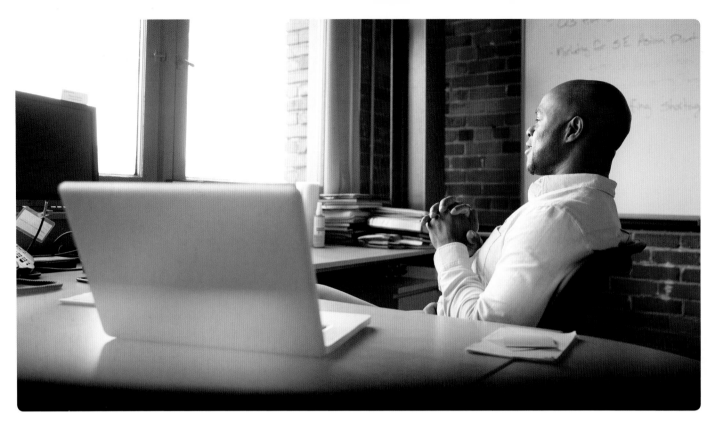

You should never feel pressured to be tested nor should you feel guilty if you decline. In the unlikely event that you find yourself facing the possibility that your baby has a genetic disorder, you will probably be offered the advantage of further counseling—an option worth serious consideration.

Finally, as in every visit to your caregiver, you will have the opportunity to bring up any concerns and questions that have come up since your last visit. Come prepared!

Your Pregnancy & Your Man

Your honey's feelings about your pregnancy may not be very obvious to you. Men tend to need time to process their emotions; they often internalize their feelings until they can come up with a way to acknowledge or express them. Your man may need a "time out" when it comes to his feelings, so give him some space, and don't push it. Also, be aware that your pregnancy may still be a bit intangible to him. After all, you don't really *look* pregnant yet, and he can't feel the baby move. The whole situation may not be on his mind as much as it is on yours, since you are the one experiencing the many physical changes that bond you with your baby.

To help your man participate in and feel connected to this pregnancy, invite him in! Think of ways to share it with him. The excitement rightfully belongs to both of you. Instead of saying "my baby" or "the baby," try "our baby." If possible, bring him along to your medical appointments. Men who go to prenatal checkups tend to have a stronger connection to the pregnancy. But even if it isn't practical for him to join you at the doctor's office, make sure to keep him up to speed on what's going on and make time to talk things through.

With some patience and understanding, your man is sure to share his feelings about becoming a father. Let him know how much you appreciate his particular ways of expressing his love to you.

Wisdom from Our Ancestors

African tribal history reveals that women were often encouraged to overcome the natural lethargy they felt during pregnancy. They were counseled to avoid oversleeping and to rise early immediately upon waking. Although they couldn't possibly have heard the term supine hypotensive syndrome—which can occur when a pregnant woman lies flat on her back, thus impeding the flow of blood through her main arteries and causing light-headedness, nausea and dizziness—women were advised to avoid this position and sleep on their sides.

Tribal women tended to be wise enough (and busy enough) to avoid sitting still for too long—something today's doctors affirm as a remedy for fainting spells and leg cramps. To prevent sagging skin and muscles, some women wore abdominal binders or belts, particularly in the later months of pregnancy or when engaged in active work.

Presently, some women wear maternity support belts during pregnancy, which is different from abdominal binders. Support belts can provide some relief for lower backache, especially during the last trimester when women experience lower back pain from increased stress on the ligaments and muscles of the lower back and spine. Abdominal binders, on the other hand, are generally worn after a woman gives birth. They are marketed as postpartum support to help women regain their shape and to look better in their clothes. There is some debate as to whether an abdominal binder has any real impact on helping a woman regain her shape. Whether it does or not, you can't discredit the fact that if a woman looks better when she puts on her clothes, she will most likely feel better. Feeling better can lead to doing more and being more active, and no one can argue the positive effects of movement.

To Do This Month

A Quick Checklist

☐ Get up slowly to avoid fainting spells.

☐ Give your man a "time out" from baby talk, if he needs it.

☐ Make a copy of the Prenatal Appointment Schedule Worksheet (page 210) and jot down your questions.

☐ Go to this month's prenatal care appointment.

CHAPTER 8

The Fourth Month

Weeks 13-16

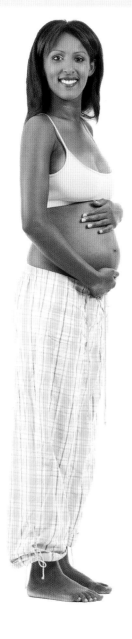

Welcome to your second trimester! This fourth month of pregnancy involves some exciting changes. You may have gained a few more pounds, but you probably feel as if someone has recharged your battery.

How You Look

Your most obvious physical change now is the growing bulge beneath your navel. Your pregnancy may now be noticeable to others, and, if you haven't already done so, you are probably having a lot of fun telling friends and family that you are expecting. And here is some more good news: your uterus is now growing up and out of your pelvic cavity and into your abdominal area, so you may not feel the need to urinate as frequently as you did in your first trimester.

Stretch Marks

Your skin is beginning to stretch over your enlarging belly and breasts, so you may see stretch marks beginning to form. These can occur when you put on weight quickly in your belly, breasts, thighs, upper arms and buttocks. They look like squiggly lines that might appear either lighter or darker than your skin tone, and they are sometimes indented or raised, almost like scars. The best way to minimize the presence of stretch marks is to gain only a healthy amount of weight during your pregnancy, and gain it slowly.

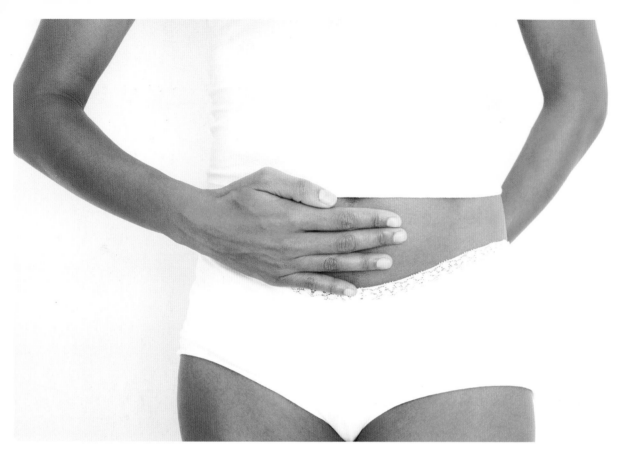

Remember, for the entire second trimester, the recommended weight gain is only 9 to 10 pounds spread over a period of 3 months. You've probably heard stories from girlfriends who gained 7 pounds in 3 weeks—but that is by no means optimal.

You might want to try moisturizing with lanolin, cocoa butter or other creams that provide some relief to the surface of the skin—but these won't prevent stretch marks. Although they bother some women, it may be psychologically healthier to accept your stretch marks as a proud badge of motherhood, not a disfigurement. And if it makes you feel better, be aware that they do tend to fade after delivery.

How You May Feel

At this point in your pregnancy, your body temperature is rising and you're probably wondering about all of that vaginal discharge. (We'll get to that a little later.) But the grandest new experience of all is feeling your baby move.

The Baby's Movements

It's called quickening, and it is one of the most significant milestones—and biggest pleasures—of pregnancy. Although the timing varies depending on your size and whether it is your first pregnancy, most women feel their babies move at the end of their fourth month or sometime during the fifth. The fluttering, bubbling sensations you feel as your baby moves around inside you are wonderful; they confirm the presence of a new life! Even though you can't yet see, hear or touch your child, you can definitely feel him now. If you don't feel any sensations of quickening by the end of your fifth month, don't panic. Discuss the fact with your practitioner.

Feeling Warm

You may begin to feel significantly warmer than usual due to increased progesterone and blood flow. Try wearing layers of clothing that can be removed when you feel uncomfortable, and indulge in cooling showers and baths when you can.

Discharge

About that discharge. Some women begin to emit a whitish substance called leukorrhea (*lu-ko-REE-a*) during this period, which increases until delivery. Although it's quite normal, it may be uncomfortable for you and a turnoff for your mate during sex. Oh well, ladies, what can we say? It's a small price to pay for the joy that's to come. Good hygiene is your best remedy. Keep your genital area clean and dry, wear soft cotton-crotch panties and change them frequently. Never use a douche without the express recommendation of your doctor—and even then, avoid a hand-bulb syringe, and never allow the bag to hang higher than about 2 feet above the level of your hips. Never insert the nozzle more than 2 inches into your vagina (or, better yet, avoid the whole operation).

Your Baby at Four Months

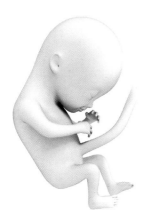

Development is dramatic and rapid for Baby now. In order to fuel this period of maximum growth, he'll need to take in a large amount of nutrients, oxygen and water, all of which are delivered by you through the placenta. At 4 months, the placenta is a little over 3 inches in diameter—a little bigger than a makeup compact. By 9 months, it will have grown to 8 inches in diameter, a bit larger than a dinner plate, and will weigh about a pound. During the fourth month, the placenta becomes a key source of hormones for you, helping your body maintain a healthy pregnancy. It also plays a big role in preparing your breasts for the production of milk.

The placenta is truly a remarkable and vital organ. It's your baby's life-support system, acting as his lungs by taking the carbon dioxide from his bloodstream and exchanging it for oxygen from yours. It acts as your baby's kidneys by filtering urine from his blood and carrying it away to your bloodstream to be eliminated through your kidneys. It also supports and regulates the transfer of iron from your circulation to your baby's.

At this stage, your baby's bones are ossifying, which means they're getting stronger. That's why you are starting to feel him move inside of you.

By the fourth month of gestation, your baby's heart has developed fully, and his pulse rate is 120 to 160 beats a minute. His spinal nerves and nerve roots have gone through myelinization (*mi-eh-lin-ih-ZAY-shun*)—an extremely important development of the nervous system. Myelin is a protective layer of fat that coats the nerves and helps convey messages to and from the brain.

By now your unborn baby's eyes have moved toward the front of his face, and he will shield them or turn away if a light shines on your belly. He can grasp his umbilical cord and suck his thumb. Taste buds have formed on his tongue, and if a bitter substance were to be injected into the amniotic fluid, he would react to it by ceasing to swallow and frowning. (Doctors have studied this!) He would react to a sweet substance the same way you might: by doubling his normal rate of ingestion.

Prenatal Care at Four Months

At this month's visit with your health-care provider, he or she will probably check the following:

- Your weight
- Your blood pressure
- Your fundal height
- The fetal heartbeat
- Your urine for sugar and protein
- Your hands and feet for swelling, and your legs for varicose veins
- Your uterine size and the growth of your baby (through abdominal palpation and measurement)

He or she will want to know if you are experiencing any unusual symptoms and will address your concerns and questions—so, as always, come prepared!

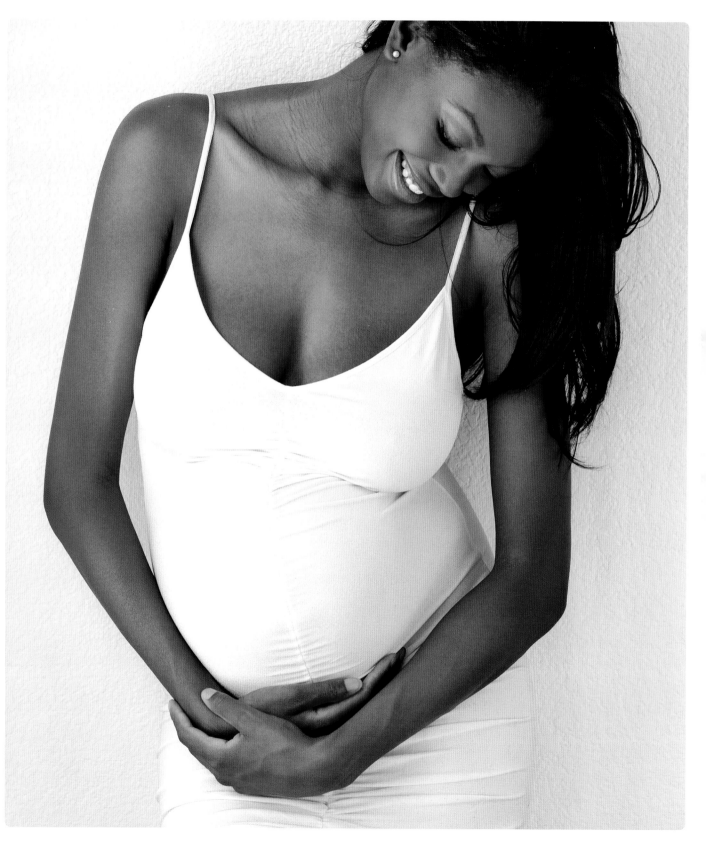

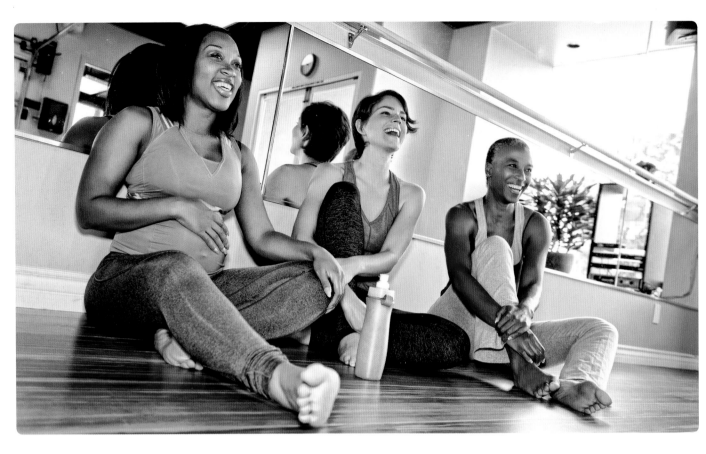

Your Pregnancy & Your Man

To maintain a healthy relationship during pregnancy, it's important for both of you to maintain your individuality and routines as well as your identity as a couple. Having a baby shouldn't mean losing your personal style or sacrificing what makes you happy—and men sometimes need reassurance of this. They need to feel secure that although many things will change when the baby comes, some things will not. You may find it useful to talk explicitly about how the two of you can continue to indulge in your private time together as well as your precious "me time" apart.

It's important to keep in mind that the challenges you face in your relationship won't disappear because you're pregnant. On the contrary, the physical, hormonal and logistical changes you are going through can magnify "hot-button" issues! Starting a family can make a good relationship great, but it can also make a shaky relationship shakier. Whatever problems you are grappling with as a couple, it is important to address them before the baby arrives—either on your own or with the help of a marriage or couples counselor. How to find the right professional? You may have a friend who can recommend someone. If not, consider contacting either the Association of Black Psychologists at 7119 Allentown Road, Suite 203, Ft. Washington, MD 20744, 301-449-3082, or the American Psychological Association at 750 First Street NE, Washington, DC, 20002-4242, 800-374-2721. These organizations can provide you with a list of therapists in your area.

Children need to grow up surrounded by adults who treat each other with love and respect and provide a loving environment for them. Please understand—by *loving* we don't mean you need to be on top of each other every moment of the day! But it is very important to create a general vibe of mutual attraction, interest, consideration, admiration and so on. Children are sponges, internalizing the principles of love based on what they experience every day—and you will be the two most important people in your baby's life. Both of you need to think about the messages your child will glean from watching you. Will he grow up understanding how a man is supposed to treat and love a woman, and how a woman is supposed to treat and love a man? These important life lessons will serve as reference points for the rest of his life as he matures, begins to connect with others and seeks out his own love relationships. Don't underestimate the importance of your child's earliest experiences of love and family.

It's worth taking a few minutes to think about how fortunate you—and your baby—are to be part of an intact family. While many of us may have been raised by single parents and live well to tell about it, studies have shown that a disproportionate number of children reared in single-family homes end up on the wrong side of the achievement gap. Specifically, children who grow up without their fathers tend to have the following:

- Less academic success
- Behavior and psychological problems
- Substance abuse problems and contact with the police
- Sexual relationships at earlier ages
- Less economic well-being in adulthood
- Less physical and psychological well-being as adults

Again, many of us are great examples of how it doesn't have to be that way. But armed with this knowledge, you and that man of yours may be inspired to reinforce your commitment to each other as a gift to the new human being you've created from love. Pledge that you will both be there for him always because you know his future depends on it. Fortify him with what he needs so that he will grow into a strong, intelligent, loving person capable of creating his own united black family. Let's obliterate this achievement gap!

Wisdom from Our Ancestors
BLACK FOLK MYTHS & SUPERSTITIONS

Between those who can't keep their hands off your belly and those who incessantly offer unsolicited advice, you might feel tempted to stay home behind a locked door. Be honored. It's just folks' way of trying to be a part of your miracle. Here are some of the gems they might impart to you—and the reality behind them:

- If you reach or stretch a lot when you're pregnant, hanging curtains for example, the baby might get strangled by the umbilical cord.

  Reality Check: Stretching your arms or reaching does nothing to your baby's umbilical cord. In fact, stretching your arms over your head exercises the muscles of the upper back, helping to relieve backache. Reaching exercises can also provide some relief if you are suffering from shortness of breath or any other breathing difficulties. Reaching expands the chest, which allows the lungs to expand to their fullest. But keep in mind that you want to be careful when reaching in general, especially during your last trimester when your center of gravity shifts. It's easier to lose your balance during the later stages of pregnancy, so standing on a chair or stool can be a dangerous business. Maybe that's where that "hanging curtains" superstition came from.

- Using a douche after intercourse will prevent pregnancy.

  Reality Check: This one couldn't be further from the truth! In fact, douching may actually increase the chances of pregnancy by pushing the sperm closer to the egg. As we mentioned in Chapter 6, a pregnant woman should never douche unless under the specific direction of her doctor. Under no circumstances should she use a hand-bulb syringe or insert the nozzle more than 2 inches into the vagina.

- When you have cramps near the end of the pregnancy, lie across your husband's belly, and the cramps will go right away.

  Reality Check: We're fairly certain no study has been done on this one! There's no harm in trying, though—and some "couple time" never hurts.

- If you crawl over your husband three times in the bed while you're pregnant, he'll get your labor pains.

  Reality Check: Let us know if this one works!

To Do This Month

A Quick Checklist

☐ Dress in layers to avoid overheating.

☐ Engage in "me time" and expect your man to do the same.

☐ Address your couple or marriage issues now.

☐ Make a copy of the Prenatal Appointment Schedule Worksheet (page 210) and jot down your questions.

☐ Go to this month's prenatal care appointment.

CHAPTER 9

The Fifth Month

Weeks 17-21

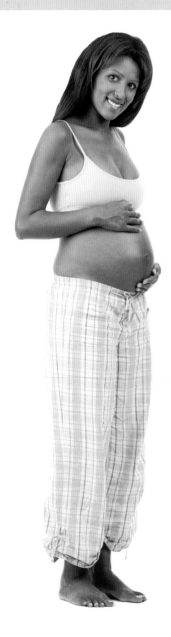

You're well into your second trimester now. Your energy is back, you're looking radiant and your body has pretty much adjusted to being pregnant. Now you can fully enjoy the experience.

How You Look

Sometime during your fifth month, or earlier for some, you may notice a change in your complexion. Your nipples are probably larger and may become darker. The line from your navel to your pubic area, called the linea nigra (*lin-AY-ah NE-grah*), may become distinctly darkened. You may also experience chloasma gravidarum, a darkening of the skin over the forehead and cheeks, which we discussed in detail back in Chapter 5. This is nothing to worry about: it's caused by high levels of estrogen and progesterone produced by the placenta, which tend to stimulate melanin production.

Those of us already blessed with beautiful brown-making melanin tend to be most affected, since deeper pigmentation changes seem to occur in women with darker complexions. There are no preventive treatments for this change, but why would you want to tamper with your beautiful brown complexion anyway? If it does concern you, try avoiding direct sunlight and use sunscreen when you're going to be outdoors in order to maintain skin health and reduce dark spots. It's important to recognize that this hyperpigmentation is a natural and harmless side effect of pregnancy, and it usually disappears after delivery.

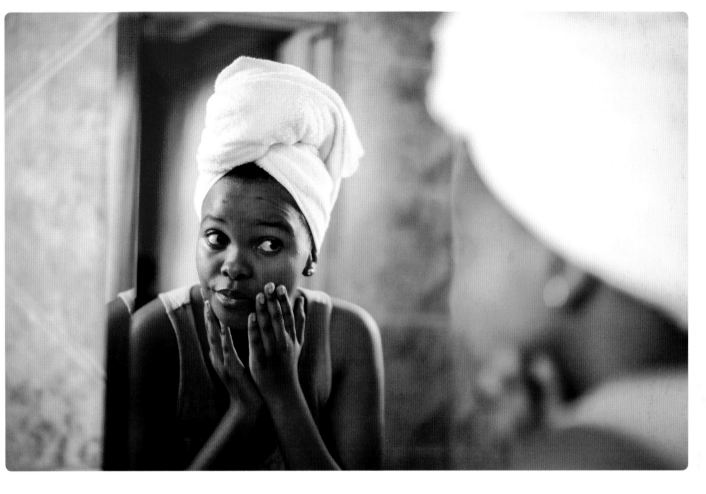

How You May Feel

Strong baby kicks and more changes in your breathing patterns are the recurring themes this month.

Your Baby's Movements

By now, your unborn baby has a strong kick and is literally turning somersaults in your womb. Since her muscles have grown larger and stronger, you may very well be able to perceive many of her activities. You may even be able to distinguish her hand from her foot and her head from her bottom. You may also become aware of her sleep and wake patterns; at this point, they are very similar to those of a newborn.

A Hyperventilating Sensation

Your growing uterus may push your diaphragm upward about 1½ inches above its normal position, which surprisingly increases its movement. This increased mobility may in turn increase the amount of air you take in and out of your lungs. More inhalations and exhalations allow for a better flow of oxygen throughout your body and more efficient removal of carbon dioxide from your bloodstream. When your carbon dioxide level gets too low, you may experience such symptoms as lightheadedness and tingling in the fingers.

An increased level of the hormone progesterone can also affect your respiratory system. Progesterone lowers carbon dioxide levels and raises oxygen levels. Between the increased mobility of your diaphragm and the effects of the increased progesterone, you may sometimes feel as if you're hyperventilating. There are no true relief measures except for the reassurance that these changes in your respiratory system are normal occurrences of pregnancy. We say that about a lot of things—but it is so true.

Dehydration

Pregnant women—especially during the first half of the pregnancy—can experience dehydration, but it can be avoided if you know what to watch out for. If your urine smells extra pungent or you have a dry mouth, you might be dehydrated.

The common cause of dehydration is nausea, as we talked about earlier. When you are nauseous and can't keep anything down, you naturally eat and drink less. This sets the stage for dehydration. Even when solid food is difficult to manage, your fluid intake is extremely important and should never be limited. If you're not able to keep fluids down, call your doctor. Depending upon how severe your condition is, he or she may send you to the emergency room for IV hydration.

Your Baby at Five Months

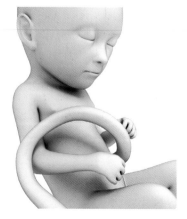

During this month, your unborn baby will grow to be about one foot tall and weigh about one pound. Fine hair will form on her eyebrows and head, along with tiny eyelashes on her still-closed eyelids. Fingernails begin to form and will probably grow until they extend beyond her fingers by the time of birth, in which case they will be in need of trimming. Her heartbeat is louder than ever, and when she's in certain positions, others can hear it by placing an ear on your belly. I'm sure her daddy will find that quite awesome.

By now her ears have moved closer to a normal position on the sides of her head. The bones within her inner ear that make hearing possible have developed and hardened, giving her the ability to hear sounds. At this point, she hears your stomach rumblings, your heart beating and her favorite sound of all, your voice.

The part of your baby's brain that is responsible for conscious thought is maturing as well, setting the stage for her to learn and remember. These great skills will be the cornerstone of her intelligence. Psychologists who used to believe that human personality was formed during the first 3 years of life now agree that it starts to take shape in the womb.

Studies show that your baby's environment and the early relationship that you and your partner develop with her can influence the formation of her personality—and that begins even before she is born. An environment that keeps your stress to a minimum is ideal. We know this is more easily said than done—especially with the addition of black stress alive and kicking in our everyday lives. But, since studies that link maternal stress to more irritable babies, it makes sense to take care of your own needs as a way to take care of her.

Research shows that black women tend to cope with stress differently from white women and men. Religion and the church have historically played a big role in helping us cope with our environment, gain insight into our lives and grapple with questions of purpose. There is also a lot to be said about spending time doing the things that you can control—and one of those is taking care of your growing baby.

Now that she can hear, your relationship with her has truly begun. You can encourage two-way communication with your baby by responding to her kicks and movements. When she kicks and moves about, try massaging your belly, creating a back-and-forth exchange with her. If she gets startled by a loud noise and kicks reflectively, rub your belly in response. Let her know all is well and Mommy is right here with her.

As your baby grows, a greasy cheese-like substance known as vernix caseosa (*VUR-neks kas-ee-Oh-sah*) begins to form a protective coating over her skin. Consisting of a combination of fatty secretions and dead skin cells, it is designed to protect your baby's delicate skin from abrasions, chapping and hardening that can result from being in amniotic fluid for so long. Lanugo (*luh-NOO-goh*), a fine woolly hair, covers her body as well. It is thought that this hair helps hold the vernix caseosa on the skin. Most of the lanugo will fall out before birth.

Although your baby's sex was determined at conception, distinctive sex organs can usually be seen by ultrasound, so if you are having this test, be sure to let the technician know whether or not you'd like to know the sex of your baby.

By the end of the fifth month, the scrotum of a male fetus is solid, and his testes will begin to descend. At 18 weeks, the uterus of a female fetus is completely formed, and her ovaries contain about 7 million eggs. (By birth, this number will be reduced to about 2 million; by adolescence she will have between 200,000 to 500,000 eggs left, of which only 400 to 500 will be released during her life.)

During the fourth and fifth months of pregnancy, your unborn baby develops the ability to produce heat and maintain her body temperature. A substance called brown fat is responsible for this important accomplishment. Deposits of brown fat can primarily be found on the unborn baby's neck, chest and crotch, and will continue to grow until birth. A lack of sufficient brown fat is one of the things that contributes to the vulnerability of premature babies. Without a sufficient amount of it, they are unable to keep themselves warm, making incubation necessary. That is also why premature babies always look so thin and frail; they haven't had a chance to develop all of their brown fat.

Since her nerve fibers are now connecting, and her limbs and muscles are stronger, your baby's movements are more deliberate and coordinated. The watery, gravity-free environment of the womb enables her to roll around and twist her spine 180 degrees, her head extending and rotating first, followed by her spine and legs. This is quite an astonishing maneuver considering that once she is born, she won't even be able to lift her own head for quite a while.

Prenatal Care at Five Months

At this month's visit with your health-care provider, he or she will probably check the following:

• Your weight

• Your blood pressure

• Your fundal height

• The fetal heartbeat

• Your urine for sugar and protein

• Your hands and feet for swelling, and your legs for varicose veins

This is the month your provider may want to perform another ultrasound. This time he or she will be conducting a head to toe scan of the baby's body parts. It's called an anatomy scan and will most likely include a look at your baby's head, heart, lungs, limbs, spine and organs. The objective is to ensure that all of your baby's body parts are growing as expected for her age.

This in-depth look at your baby will also include an analysis of your cervical length. The focus on your cervix is important because doctors can determine whether you are at risk for preterm birth by the length of your cervix. It may be uncomfortable to think about such complications, especially since you and the baby are probably doing fine; however, so much more can be done successfully when doctors can foresee a potential problem. And that's what you want, a plan to keep you and your baby healthy for the duration of your pregnancy, rather than a reaction to an emergency.

Your doctor will want to know if you are experiencing any unusual symptoms and will address your concerns and questions—so, as always, come prepared!

Planning Baby's Birthday

Around this time, you might start thinking more about the birth itself and decide what kind of birth experience you want to have. Pregnant women often have a number of questions regarding labor and childbirth, with the most frequent question being, "Can someone else do it for me?" While that's not possible, you do have some choices when it comes to managing your labor and childbirth, and this is a good time to start educating yourself on your options.

Though the process of giving birth is accomplished in only one of three ways—natural childbirth, medically supported vaginal birth or cesarean section—the experience itself is as varied as the millions of women who go through it every year. Your second birth experience won't even be the same as your first. So let's just get to what's probably on your mind: the pain. The truth is that the amount of discomfort and pain you experience during childbirth depends on a few factors, including the size of the baby, her position, the strength of your contractions and your pain tolerance.

Natural childbirth offers many benefits, as does taking advantage of all that modern medicine has to offer. And it's possible to opt for the best of both worlds, incorporating aspects of natural childbirth with some medical interventions. Keep in mind that there is no wrong or right way to birth your baby. Remember that the purpose of the whole experience is to be able to see and touch that beautiful little brown face at the end of the day. (Well, maybe not so brown at first; it often takes some time for the melanin to kick in.)

Prior to the rise of the natural childbirth movement, professionals and laypeople alike looked upon pregnancy as a medical procedure. The pregnant woman was a patient, and the doctor was the sole decision maker. Ensuring the physical safety of mother and baby was the only priority of business during childbirth, exclusive of the mother's emotional and psychological needs. Today, the fields of obstetrics and gynecology have responded to women's desire to be an active participant in the birthing process.

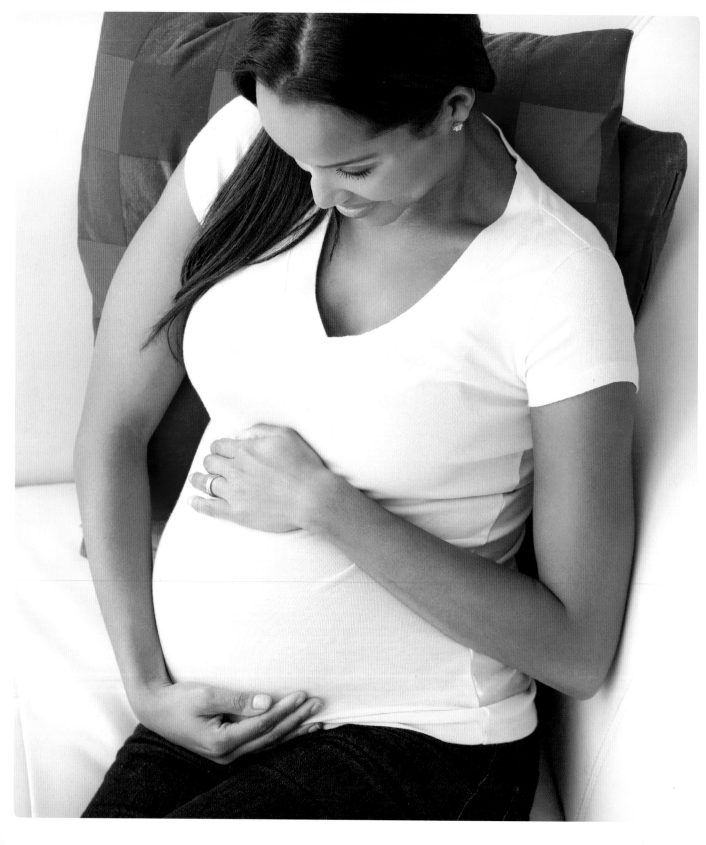

Just because you might want to give birth in a hospital with medical professionals standing by doesn't mean the process is out of your hands. In most hospitals, procedures can been adapted to meet your needs as well as your baby's, and you are likely to be consulted more fully at every turn. At this point, we don't think anyone would disagree with the notion that a successful birth experience is one in which the physical well-being of mother and baby are achieved as well as a sense of emotional fulfillment for both parents. You can now honestly say to yourself, "I am an empowered woman, I know I have choices, and I play an active role in the birth of my child. No one delivers my baby for me; *I* deliver my child with assistance." These are very strong statements and can do wonders for your self-esteem and feelings of self-sufficiency—and rightfully so. This is one of those rare moments in your life when you've earned the right to feel like the most important person in the world.

Considering Natural Childbirth

Many people feel that choosing natural childbirth helps make this major event a more satisfying experience. But, what is natural childbirth exactly?

In natural childbirth, labor and birth are considered a normal and healthy process that under routine circumstances needs no medical intervention.

Proponents argue that laboring women shouldn't be seen as patients in need of medical intervention since our bodies are completely capable of delivering babies into the world as part of their normal functioning. There must be something to this concept, because it's pretty much all our great-great-grandmothers had to rely on when they gave birth, and they managed to produce and maintain a strong black race. If you want to consider natural childbirth today, it's important to be informed and prepared about what exactly happens during the birth process and ways to cooperate with and tune in to your body's inner wisdom.

You should also know that people interpret "natural childbirth" to mean different things. At one extreme are those who believe that a truly natural labor and birth involve no use of drugs like an epidural, to ease pain, or medical interventions such as forceps or vacuums to facilitate birth. Yet there are others who believe that whenever a woman delivers vaginally, it is natural childbirth regardless of the type of intervention she needed. According to this perspective, a woman could be medicated with an intravenous needle in her arm, attached to electronic fetal monitors and confined to a bed, and still have natural childbirth.

Who Can Have Natural Childbirth

If you choose to have a drug-free birth with no medical interventions, you can do so as long as you're not at risk for any complications. Your pregnancy must be proceeding normally, and you must have the physical endurance to manage such a process. It's important that you start early in your pregnancy to learn how to help yourself mentally and physically during labor.

Why Choose Natural Childbirth?

Many women choose natural childbirth because they are aware that conventional birth practices sometimes increase their dependency on medical intervention rather than rely on their own body's natural functioning. For example, medical doctors are concerned that a laboring woman might regurgitate and inhale vomit if general anesthesia is needed and used during labor. In order to avoid this dangerous situation, no food or drink by mouth is usually the rule in case the need for anesthesia arises. However, not eating or drinking during a time of great strenuous activity could cause the woman to become dehydrated. So to avoid dehydration, the laboring woman is hooked up to an IV. Unfortunately, an IV makes it difficult for the woman to move into the positions that she may feel most comfortable in. Inactivity can and often does prolong labor. Think about it for a second. What acts do you think will most likely facilitate labor and birth: getting up from the bed, walking around or squatting (with gravity helping the baby through the birth canal) or lying in bed semi-upright? Once a woman is limited to a bed and hooked up to an IV, labor can slow down to the point where the doctor may need to intervene with medications to speed things up. This is just one example of how one type of medical intervention could lead to dependency on another. Opting to use more natural childbirth methods when possible can help prevent this chain of events.

Methods of Natural Childbirth

There are a number of special techniques, procedures and philosophies for facilitating natural childbirth. Most of these methods have more similarities than differences. Whatever method you choose, you will most likely find information about labor and birth, ways of relaxing and releasing muscle tension, breathing exercises and physical conditioning techniques. Here are some of the leading types:

- **Certified nurse midwife (CNM).** Pregnancy, labor and birth are all supported by CNMs, who believe in treating pregnancy and a baby's birth as a normal, healthy process. They pride themselves on providing vigilant and attentive care, intervening minimally and only when required. Opting for a midwife-attended birth means you will have the opportunity to make decisions about your pregnancy and baby's birth. A CNM can help you deliver in a hospital, where he or she works collaboratively with hospital staff, as well as in a birthing center or at home. CNMs offer you continued care after the baby is born and throughout your life span if you desire.

- **Water birth.** This one always seems a little hard for us to wrap our heads around at first because of the concept of a precious newborn submerged in water. However, we have to remember while in the womb, a baby never takes air into her lungs. Her oxygen supply comes straight from Mother in the form of rich, oxygenated blood through the umbilical cord. It's not until a newborn is exposed to air that the instinct to take a breath occurs. This type of introduction to the world is thought to be far more calming and gentler for a baby than the seemingly harsher bright lights, louder noise and colder temperature of a labor room birth.

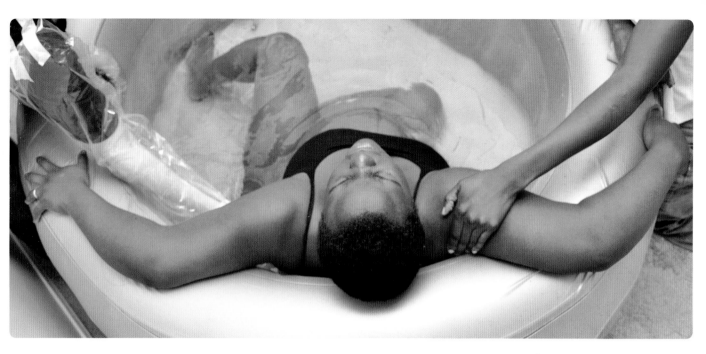

For the laboring mom, the buoyancy of warm water can be very relaxing, which certainly helps in pain management. Relaxing muscles so that contractions can really do their job moving the baby down through the cervix helps to create a more effective labor and birth experience. Some women just labor in water then exit the tub for the actual delivery. Some, of course, choose to give birth in the water. There are a number of hospitals with birthing tubs, thereby making water births an option for more women. However, not every doctor is convinced that it is safe. You can have a water birth in a hospital or a birthing center, or you can choose to deliver in a bathtub in a home birth. Having qualified, experienced and well-trained health-care providers assist you is an absolute necessity. It's also important to know that water births are not recommended for women experiencing a high-risk pregnancy, if the baby is in a breech position (bottom or feet down) or if you are having any complications in general with your pregnancy. If you are seriously thinking about a water birth, commit a good amount of time to researching the benefits as well as the risks associated with this method of childbirth.

- **Home birth.** This method is considered the ultimate natural childbirth method, as it most resembles what would naturally happen in the laboring woman's life. It is how our great-great-grandmothers delivered our ancestors into the world. Essentially, home births are drug-free births that allow a laboring woman to remain in the comfort and familiarity of her home while her body engages in the business of bringing forth a new human being. The great benefit here is the autonomy you can have regarding your labor and baby's birth. Certainly the lighting, temperature and sounds, along with who comes and goes throughout the experience, are based primarily on your needs and wants. Again it goes without saying that it is important to have a certified, experienced and well-trained health-care provider with you to assist in this birthing experience.

- **Lamaze.** This method has been around a little longer than some of the other methods and is a little more widely recognized. It seems to have evolved from a specific method of childbirth that focused on distraction techniques and breathing, to a philosophy that focuses on educating women and guiding them as they prepare to give birth. The Lamaze Healthy Birth Practices include the following:
  - Let labor begin on its own
  - Walk, move around and change positions throughout labor
  - Bring a loved one or friend for continuous support
  - Avoid interventions that are not medically necessary
  - Avoid giving birth on your back and follow your body's urges to push
  - Keep mother and baby together—it's best for mother, baby and breast-feeding

- **The Bradley method.** This method focuses on the couple or family and teaches them that natural childbirth techniques are based on information about how the human body works during labor. Couples are taught how they can work with their bodies to reduce pain and make their labors more efficient. They also stress the importance of natural childbirth without the side effects of drugs given during labor and birth. They offer 12-week classes, which are taken during the last 3 months—your last trimester of pregnancy. Physical exercises are taught along with information on labor and birth, relaxation and nutrition. Dr. Bradley, an American OB-GYN in the late 1940s, developed this method and compared birth to swimming. In summary, his point is that if someone threw you in 10 feet of water at the end of 9 months of pregnancy, it could be very scary for you. And if you didn't know how to swim, you could even drown or would have to be saved by a lifeguard. However, if you took the time to take classes and learn how to swim, that experience could end quite differently, hence the need for preparation classes.

- **The Leboyer method.** Leboyer involves creating a birthing atmosphere that's less harsh on the newborn's senses. It's not a method of preparation for birth, but rather a method of greeting the newborn in a gentle and sensitive manner. Dr. Frédérick Leboyer presents a picture in his book *Birth without Violence* of what truly appears to be a very harsh beginning for a newly born baby. He describes a newborn's experience of being pulled out of the birth canal with forceps, held up to be shown to mother, drained of mucus, having its cord cut and then being placed on a hard surface under glaring lights. Those traditional procedures he felt constituted unnecessarily harsh treatment of the baby, so he substituted a more sensitive approach. In the Leboyer method, lights are dimmed, noise is kept to a minimum, and the newborn is immediately placed in warm water with the umbilical cord intact before its full introduction to the world. The baby is massaged, offered the opportunity to nurse and be cuddled, often skin to skin.

- **The Mongan method.** If you are a fan of hypnotism, then this just might be the method for you. Marie Mongan, certified hypnotherapist, wrote a book on HypnoBirthing in 1989. This method teaches women self-hypnosis techniques designed to create total relaxation to let the laboring body do what is needed. Supporters of this method believe that the majority of birthing women do not need interventions or procedures for safe and healthy births. Nor do they think women need special exercises or scripts for childbirth preparation. The Mongan method focuses mothers on programming their minds and conditioning their bodies to birth easily. Trained health-care providers called hynotherapists assist the laboring woman with being extremely focused and using endorphins released in the brain to help block pain. Once the pain is blocked, muscles can relax, thereby allowing the laboring body to do what it will naturally do: push the baby through her birth path.

Considering Childbirth with Medication

Despite the benefits of choosing what's considered purely natural childbirth, many women still feel reassured with the high-tech medical procedures available in hospitals. Many opt for some form of medication during labor and childbirth. Some women proudly proclaim, "I'm not trying to be a hero. Why shouldn't I take advantage of pain relief medication when it's safe for me and my baby?" And they're absolutely right to think that way. It actually makes you just as empowered as the "birth without medication" moms. It really is all about you, your body, your baby and your family. It's about what you want and what you don't want, and as long as you have the right conditions, it's about getting just that.

To help you cope better with your pain, there are a number of drugs that are available. You can plan to use pain relief medication during labor in a very logical manner as long as you understand the various drugs that are used, their effects and the condition under which they are administered. It's best to find out as much as possible about them beforehand, so talk with your doctor about your pain relief concerns and preferences early on. Don't be too rigid with what you want and what you don't want, since you really won't know what your pain tolerance is until you're actually going through it. Skip ahead to Chapter 14 for a full description of the pain relief medication available for the laboring woman.

Whether you want and plan for a natural childbirth or one with medication, know that complications can and do completely change the birthing process into a more medically oriented management. By being well prepared and cooperating with your doctor during a medical complication or emergency, you can give informed consent to procedures even though your physician is the primary decision maker.

In all honesty, whenever a woman gives birth, it's a natural experience regardless of how it occurs. The type of birthing experience you have is going to be very much individualized. Every woman has her own unique attitude, beliefs, particular ways of moving, previous medical history, genetic makeup and approach to the medical world. All of these important variables play a role in the experience of birth.

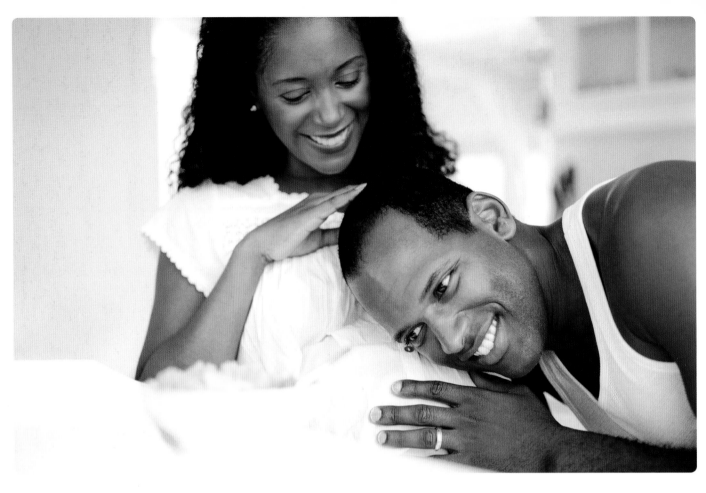

Your Pregnancy & Your Man

At this stage in your pregnancy, your baby can hear some sounds, so now more than ever, what she hears is what she may connect with easiest after birth. Although your voice, heartbeat and the gurgling sounds of your digestion may pretty much dominate what she hears, her daddy's voice can and should be a constant as well. It's important that her daddy knows he can communicate with his baby, too. And communication is not limited to just talking. Actually, communication is about relaying and receiving messages, and it doesn't matter how the message is sent. You and your partner can pat your stomach, dance together, talk to, sing to and massage your baby now, all of which communicates love and nurturance. And let's not forget about music. With your unborn baby's ability to hear, now you and your partner can use music as a wonderful medium for connecting with her. Music with a tempo of 60 to 70 beats per minute is similar to that of the resting human heartbeat. This kind of tempo can be calming for the baby, as well as for you and her daddy. If you and your man listen to music often enough and allow it to soothe you, it just may have that same effect on all of you when you go into labor. Labor is obviously a time when the three of you would need soothing the most.

Music is great, but if it's not for you and your honey, don't worry. The power of words and plain old talking is just as effective or better. There are countless stories by women who swear their unborn baby moves, shifts or just becomes more alert when their partner walks in and speaks to them. We don't doubt this for a second, which is all the more reason why talking to your unborn baby now creates and reinforces your special bond as a family.

Wisdom from Our Ancestors

A FLASHBACK IN TIME

There is a tribe in Africa where the birth date of a child is counted not from when they've been born, nor from when they are conceived but from the day that the child was a thought in its mother's mind.

And when a woman decides that she will have a child, she goes off and sits under a tree by herself, and she listens until she can hear the song of the child that wants to come. And after she's heard the song of this child, she comes back to the man who will be the child's father, and teaches it to him. And then, when they make love to physically conceive the child, some of that time they sing the song of the child, as a way to invite it.

And then, when the mother is pregnant, the mother teaches that child's song to the midwives and the old women of the village, so that when the child is born, the old women and the people around her sing the child's song to welcome it. And then, as the child grows up, the other villagers are taught the child's song. If the child falls, or hurts its knee, someone picks it up and sings its song to it. Or perhaps the child does something wonderful, or goes through the rites of puberty, and then as a way of honoring this person, the people of the village sing his or her song.

And it goes this way through their life. In marriage, the songs are sung, together. And finally, when this child is old and lying in bed, ready to die, all the villagers know his or her song, and they sing—for the last time—the song to that person.

Somé, Sobonfu. *Welcoming Spirit Home: Ancient African Teachings to Celebrate Children and Community.* Novato, California: New World Library, 1999

That really gives new meaning to "it takes a village to raise a child."

To Do This Month

A Quick Checklist

☐ Avoid sunlight if you are experiencing chloasma gravidarum.

☐ Talk to your baby; she can hear you now.

☐ Start thinking about your expectations for your labor and your baby's birthday experience.

☐ Remind your honey to talk to his baby.

☐ Make a copy of the Prenatal Appointment Schedule Worksheet (page 210) and jot down your questions.

☐ Go to this month's prenatal care appointment.

CHAPTER 10

The Sixth Month

Weeks 22-26

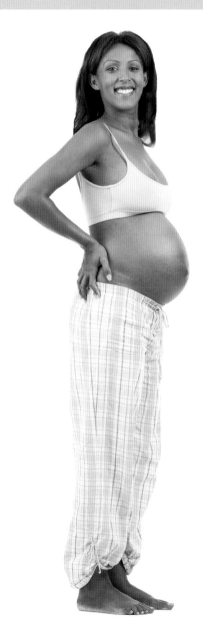

You're six months pregnant and looking great, Mom! Your pregnancy should continue to bring many changes, including some pleasant surprises.

How You Look

Your face is probably looking fuller, mostly due to the excess water your body is retaining. You're gaining more weight now, and your belly is growing rapidly. Your hair is also probably growing longer and fuller—a nice perk of pregnancy.

Let's take this opportunity to talk a bit more about our hair during pregnancy because—let's face it—as beautiful black women, we pay a lot of attention to our hair! Leslie Louard-Davis, former hair salon owner for over 26 years and current educator, advises that a good hair maintenance program during pregnancy should include weekly shampoos and conditioning. If you find that your hair is becoming dry, you'll want to be diligent in keeping it moisturized. Natural oils, coconut and olive oils (extra virgin), in conjunction with your weekly conditioners are effective measures against dry, brittle hair. Davis also suggests that you be aware of perspiration. When you sweat, your sebaceous glands secrete salt, which has a drying effect on hair. So if you tend to perspire a lot in general or if a sweat-inducing exercise regimen is part of your routine, you may need to wash and condition your hair more than once a week.

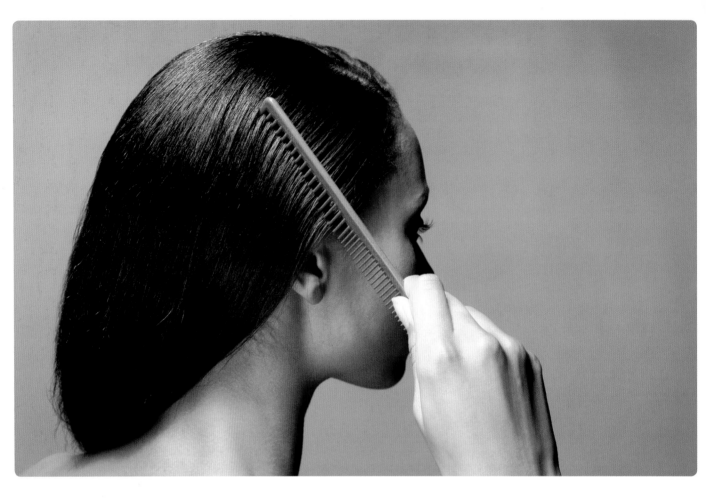

Oily hair requires shampooing even more frequently than once a week, preferably with a shampoo formulated specifically for oily hair, which can be purchased at your local drugstore or salon.

Now for the big question: should you continue to get touch-ups during your pregnancy? Dr. Sumayah Jamal states that there is little evidence to support that chemical relaxers have adverse effects on the developing fetus. She goes on to state that minimal amounts of relaxer ingredients are absorbed through the scalp, and in general there is a lack of toxicity in those ingredients. She warns, though, if you have wounds, scratches or burns of the scalp prior to your touch-up, you can increase the absorption of the relaxer. So if your scalp is not free of scratches or wounds, you should not get a touch-up. The almighty base coat is an important step in the process because it minimizes the chance of your scalp being burned by the chemicals. Additionally, Dr. Jamal warns that you should be getting your touch-up in a well-ventilated area to disperse the fumes, which can cause nausea or headaches.

Keratin hair straighteners are a different story, however. Jamal states that the use of keratin straighteners is discouraged during pregnancy due to the inclusion of formaldehyde in their ingredients or the release of formaldehyde when the preparation is exposed to heat. She adds that formaldehyde is readily absorbed by skin and is also toxic.

In regard to hair coloring during pregnancy, Dr. Jamal states that as with relaxers, there is little evidence of systemic absorption of the dyes, and there is a general lack of toxicity in those ingredients. She goes on to suggest using highlights if you are really concerned, since the coloring is applied to the hair shaft only. Using hair-coloring products with natural vegetable dyes is another alternative for women who prefer to stay on the safer side.

How You May Feel

This month brings wonderful things. By the end of it, you'll be able to share with your honey and others the indescribable sensation of your unborn baby moving inside you because his kicks will have grown so strong that they will be easy for loved ones to feel! On the downside, you might also come face-to-face with some less happy side effects.

Heartburn

During the sixth month of pregnancy, it's common for women to experience heartburn—and not because the baby has a lot of hair, as some old wives' tales would lead you to believe! Your heartburn is a result of the crowding inside your body. Your little one, who is growing bigger by the day, is pressing against and shifting your stomach, and this can cause your stomach acid to back up into your esophagus and throat. Cue the burning sensation. Adding insult to injury, heartburn is exacerbated by the increase in progesterone in your body, which relaxes the smooth muscles and delays the emptying of the acidic digestive juices from your stomach.

What's a woman to do? To lessen the discomforts of heartburn, have small, frequent meals rather than fewer, larger ones as a way to avoid overloading your stomach. You may also want to do the following:

- Avoid excessively fatty meals since fat tends to slow down stomach movement and the secretion of digestive juices.
- Avoid very cold foods, which also tend to slow down the digestive process.
- Drink cultured milk (buttermilk vs. sweet milk) between meals if you find it tolerable, although this obviously doesn't apply if, like many of us, you are lactose intolerant.
- Maintain good posture, since this gives your stomach more room to function optimally.
- Remain in an upright position for three to four hours after eating, and definitely avoid bending over immediately after a meal.
- Take low-sodium antacids if your health-care practitioner feels you are a candidate for them.

Constipation

Some women experience the discomfort of constipation during pregnancy. Again, the culprit is the hormone progesterone, which causes the smooth muscles, those responsible for moving wastes out of the system, to become relaxed. Your enlarging uterus also contributes to the unpleasantness, since it's putting pressure upon and displacing your intestines. All of this can result in constipation—and relief begins with good bowel habits.

Attempt a bowel movement at the same time each day, but be careful not to strain too much, since that can cause hemorrhoids. Make sure your diet includes high-fiber foods that will stimulate peristalsis (*per-eh-STAHL-sis*)—the movement of waste through your intestines—and soften your stool. High-fiber foods include cereal products such as bran, whole-grain bread, fruit, vegetables and legumes. Drinking warm liquids in the morning may also provide some relief, as will regular exercise. As always, make sure you talk to your provider prior to starting any exercise routine.

Gas

As if constipation weren't bad enough on its own, a side "benefit" is that when your intestinal tract is sluggish and waste remains in your body for a prolonged period, the bacteria in your intestines ferment, causing gas. The change in the position of your intestines and the pressure exerted on them by your uterus also contribute to the problem. For relief, pay attention to what you eat. Avoid large meals and fatty and gas-forming foods such as onions and beans. Frequent exercise may also help. For all intestinal problems, it's important to maintain regular bowel function; see the section above on constipation for ways to ensure this.

Changes in Your Heart Rate

It's common during the second trimester for a woman to feel a change in her heart rate. You may notice arrhythmia, a momentary rhythm disruption that many women describe as "skipping a beat," sensing extra beats, or just a momentary feeling of pressure in the neck and chest area. In fact, the average pregnant woman's heart rate does increase by 10 to 20 beats per minute. Some women even develop a heart murmur. Rest assured that these changes are usually benign and do not indicate that you are developing heart disease. They are primarily caused by the extra demands put on your heart and circulatory system in supporting your baby's life as well as your own. Although these sensations may frighten you when they occur, they are no real threat to either of you. When you sense an arrhythmia, try coughing or taking a deep breath to convert your heart rate back to a more normal pattern. And, of course, be sure to mention these events to your practitioner so that he or she always has a complete picture of your pregnancy as it unfolds. Your heart will return to its normal routine after pregnancy.

Swelling

If you haven't suffered from swollen feet and ankles yet, don't be surprised if you do so now. The increase in the amount of blood the pregnant body produces and the decrease in its speed of circulation combine to cause swelling in many women. But there are additional factors, too. High salt intake and water retention caused by the hormones of pregnancy are just as guilty in causing those swollen feet and ankles. So if ever there was the perfect time to train your taste buds into liking less salty foods, it's now. If you haven't already, try some of the tasty recipes in Chapter 2 that were created with you in mind: soulful meals made with less salt and fat but full of flavor.

So you are monitoring your salt intake, but your feet keep outgrowing your shoes. What can you do? Elevating your feet and legs for a time throughout the day may improve your circulation and reduce the swelling somewhat. Also, be sure to get sufficient rest and avoid clothing that binds, such as garters or tight pants and socks. When sleeping or lying down, try to stay on your left side, thus preventing your uterus from blocking adequate blood flow from your heart. Also, make sure you get enough water: at least eight glasses a day.

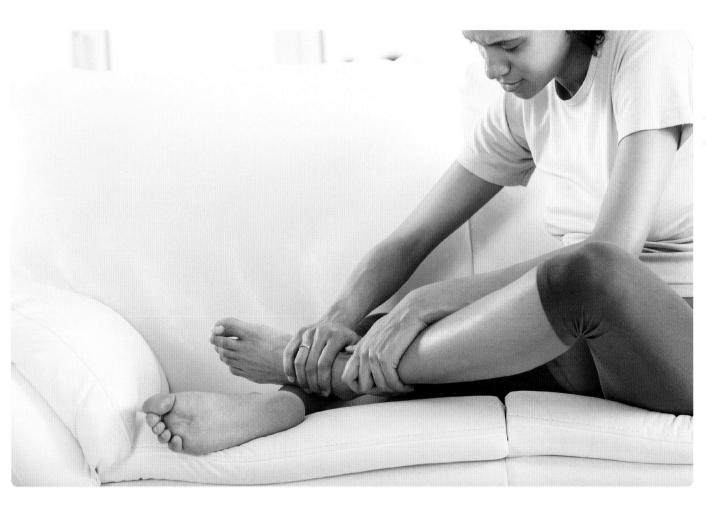

Your Baby at Six Months

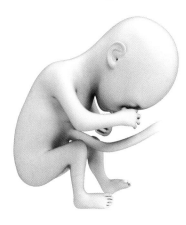

During month six, your unborn baby will grow about 2 more inches to become about 14 inches long. He will also gain a significant amount of weight—about 1.75 pounds—and begin to accumulate a little fat under his skin. Buds for permanent teeth will come in high in his gums, behind his baby teeth. Since his eyelids can now open, he may open and close them and look up, down and sideways.

Another important milestone is the development of a substance called surfactant (*ser-FAK-tent*), which will eventually make it possible for your baby to breathe on his own. Surfactant keeps the small air sacs in the lungs, called alveoli, slightly inflated. Why is this important? Just as it's easier to blow up a balloon that has already been inflated somewhat, when the big time comes for Baby to breathe on his own, it won't be so difficult. His respiratory system is actually practicing for that day. His nostrils have now opened, and he may make breathing motions. When babies are born prematurely, they often lack sufficient surfactant and must undergo surfactant replacement therapy.

You will be delighted to find that your baby can now listen and respond to what he hears. He will move his body in sync with your speech, a behavior that will continue after he is born. Wow—how precious is that?

Prenatal Care at Six Months

At this month's visit with your health-care provider, he or she will probably check the following:

- Your weight
- Your blood pressure
- Your fundal height
- The fetal heartbeat
- Your urine for sugar and protein
- Your hands and feet for swelling, and your legs for varicose veins
- Your uterine size and the growth of your baby (through abdominal palpation and measurement)

As always, come prepared with your questions and concerns.

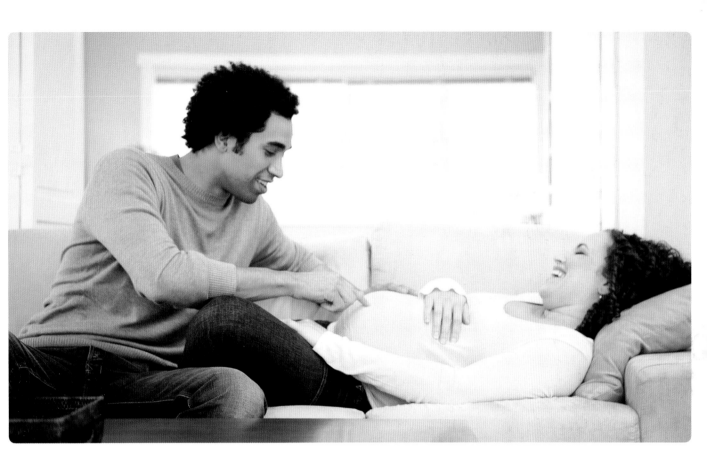

Your Pregnancy & Your Man

We can't stress enough the importance of good, open communication between you and your sweetheart throughout this huge life transition—especially now that your body is changing profoundly. Just as you are becoming accustomed to the physical changes going on, you want him to be comfortable and familiar with those changes as well. Pick a time when you are both relaxed and encourage him to look at and explore the contours of your ever-changing body.

In Chapter 4, we discussed some massage techniques you can share, but now a different kind of touch is called for. The objective here is to give your guy the opportunity to connect physically with his unborn baby. Guiding his hands and encouraging him, let him discover where the baby is inside of you and what position he is in. Let him feel those kicks and flips. Besides helping him feel closer to his child, this experience may help him understand the toll that pregnancy is taking on you. It is important for you to connect in this way because you are a threesome now. (And if this exploration session leads to something a bit more sensual and you're both in the mood for it, there's no harm in that!)

Wisdom from Our Ancestors

BLACK FOLK MYTHS & SUPERSTITIONS

BABY TRAITS & MARKS

Oh, boy! The last thing you need is the guilt of knowing your child has to live with a big birthmark on his forehead in the shape of a fish because you went a little overboard with Goldfish crackers when you were pregnant. These days, not many of us believe the old superstitions about diet during pregnancy. Still, it's fun to hear them, so here are some golden oldies that are probably still circulating:

- If you crave something when you're pregnant and you eat a lot of it, your baby will have a mark that looks like the thing you craved.
- You should never laugh at someone's looks during pregnancy or your child will be born looking like that person.
- If you experience a lot of heartburn while pregnant, your baby will have a lot of hair.

As we discussed, heartburn is a result of digestive problems that often occur when the uterus begins to push on the stomach. It has nothing to do with hair quantity or quality, which are determined by genetics.

- If you see anything that scares you or makes you sad, it will mark the baby; therefore, horror movies and funerals are to be avoided.

Well . . . you do want to try to stay calm and happy for the sake of your baby—so perhaps there is a kernel of truth in this one. But we do know that the connection between your own distress and your baby's is a bit more physical and less mystical.

- It's bad luck to buy clothes for the baby before the baby's born. It is, however permissible for others to buy things ahead of time for the baby and give them to you at a baby shower.

We know lots of women who feel superstitious about buying things ahead of time—as if they are tempting fate by assuming that all will go according to plan. If it makes you feel better to wait, by all means do it. You might want to have large items such as a crib or changing table stored unopened in your garage or basement. But we can't endorse the scientific veracity of this superstition. The best way to ensure that you will have a healthy baby is to stay on top of your prenatal care throughout your pregnancy.

- If your baby is born with holes in his ears (usually where the top of the ear joins the head), he will be able to foresee the future—but only during childhood.
- Similarly, if your baby is born with a veil, or caul, he will be able to see the future.

When the amniotic sac doesn't break during labor or delivery, the baby may be born fully encased in it. This membrane is the caul. The situation is perfectly normal, causes no risk to the baby—and doesn't mean he's a little fortune-teller.

To Do This Month

A Quick Checklist

☐ Keep hair moisturized.

☐ Eat frequent but small meals to avoid heartburn.

☐ Eat high-fiber foods to avoid constipation.

☐ Cough if you are sensing a change in your heart rate.

☐ Reduce your salt intake.

☐ Make a copy of the Prenatal Appointment Schedule Worksheet (page 210) and jot down your questions.

☐ Go to this month's prenatal care appointment.

CHAPTER 11

The Seventh Month

Weeks 27-30

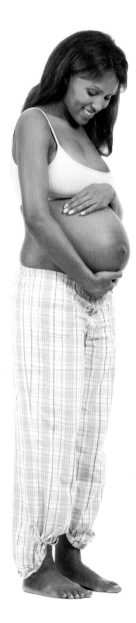

Congratulations! You have finally made it to your last trimester. This is a very exciting time in your pregnancy—one that's filled with lots of emotion.

How You Look

By now you will have gained a good amount of weight, so you are "showing," and your pregnancy is certainly having an impact on your day-to-day activities.

Don't be surprised to find milk leaking from your nipples at this stage. Yep, this can happen at certain times, such as when warm water hits them in the shower or when you're sexually aroused. It's because your body is beginning to produce colostrum, the fluid that precedes true breast milk. You may want to try a well-fitted nursing bra during these last months of pregnancy. The pads that go in a nursing bra, which you can buy in the baby section of most drug stores, will prevent the colostrum from staining your clothes. By the end of this month, you will probably have gained a total of 2 to 3 pounds in breast weight, and your breasts will be at their maximum pregnancy size (but they are likely to grow a bit more once your baby is born and lactation starts, which is your milk production process). This means you'll need to go up at least a cup size to accommodate the increased fullness of your breasts.

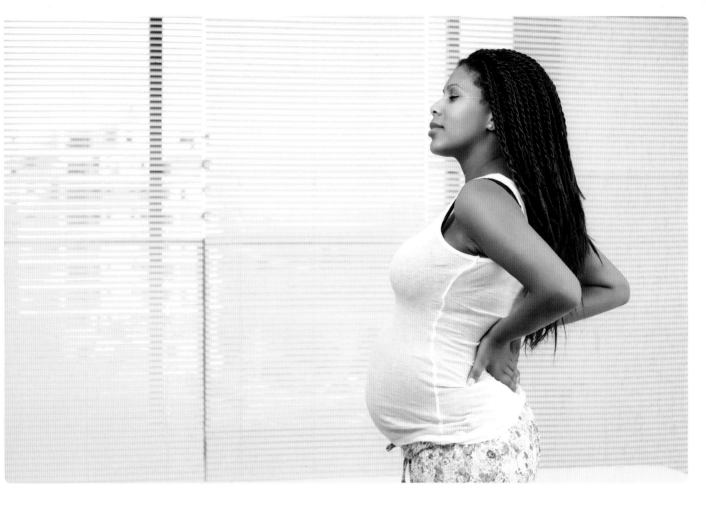

How You May Feel

Now that you've entered your last three months of pregnancy, you are likely to encounter new physical challenges and limitations.

Backache

As your growing baby extends your belly forward, your center of gravity moves forward as well. To compensate, you'll tend to lean backward for better balance, creating that classic pregnancy stance in your back. As you can imagine, this puts quite a strain on the muscles and ligaments of your lower back. It doesn't help that your body has increased its production of relaxin, a hormone that helps soften your ligaments in preparation for labor and birth. Softer ligaments are a good thing when it comes time to push a baby out of your body, but right now they can be less effective in supporting the weight of your developing fetus.

How to relieve that pregnancy backache? Safe, regular exercise—including walking, swimming and riding a stationary bike—will help strengthen your lower back muscles. But be sure to consult with your health-care provider before starting any exercise routine. You may also want to talk to him or her about applying hot or cold compresses to your aches and pains. Both temperatures have the potential to make you feel better, but be careful to keep hot packs away from your belly.

You should also be mindful of your posture, which can have a profound effect on your back at any time but especially during pregnancy. Avoid slouching, which places a strain on your spine. When seated, try to keep your back straight and elevate your feet slightly with a stool, which should provide immediate relief to your back and shoulders. You might even want to try a support belt, especially if your daily routine involves a lot of moving around.

Fatigue

Fatigue returns during these last months, primarily because of the increased work your heart is doing as you carry around the extra weight of baby. Fatigue is your body's way of telling you to slow down—advice you should always try to take. You may find it necessary to shorten your activity periods and take more time for rest.

Ambivalent Feelings

Feelings of ambivalence may surge again as you come within 12 weeks of the birth of your baby. On the one hand, you can hardly wait to see her; but on the other hand, you may also feel unready for parenthood or for another baby in your life. One moment you may be in awe of the pregnancy experience and delighted by your growing belly, the next you may feel anxious about those extra pounds and the fact that your body is out of your control.

Your work may be weighing heavily on your mind, too, as you face maternity leave and the impact it may have on your family's financial stability. Plus, there is the extra burden your coworkers will have to shoulder. Rest assured that you are not alone in your concerns. Most women experience an emotional roller coaster during this time, but few problems are insurmountable, especially with the love and support of your mate, family and friends. Share your concerns with them, try to enjoy the last few months of your pregnancy and don't allow the stress of it all to get to you.

Breathing Difficulties

You may be experiencing a stuffy nose. Hormonal increases and extra blood flow cause swelling of the mucous membranes that line your nose. That, along with the pressure of your growing uterus on your diaphragm, can make breathing harder. "Reaching" exercises may provide some relief, as the expansion of your chest improves the efficiency of your respiratory system. Simply extend your arms up and over your head whenever you have trouble breathing. Contrary to old folk beliefs, this will not cause the umbilical cord to twist around your baby's neck. As for the stuffiness, try taking a warm shower or bath; the steam can be soothing and can relieve some of the congestion.

Back to the Bathroom

OMG! Here we go again. As in the first trimester, you may once again find yourself making frequent trips to the bathroom. As your baby grows and "engages" her way down into your pelvic area—right next to your bladder—you may feel the need to urinate often. As you did during your first trimester, you should try to drink most of your liquids during the day, tapering off toward bedtime in order to limit interruptions when you're trying to sleep. Never restrict fluids drastically, of course, and always answer nature's call. "Holding it" can lead to a urinary tract infection, and that's the last thing you need right now.

Hemorrhoids

Hemorrhoids—itchy or painful masses of swollen veins near or just inside of your anus—can be vexing at this time, too. Pressure from your enlarging uterus, specifically on the hemorrhoidal veins (those by your rectum), can cause this condition. Preventing constipation can help ward off hemorrhoids, since straining while having a bowel movement is a contributing factor. So, as we discussed in Chapter 10, drink plenty of fluids, eat fiber-rich foods and establish regular bowel habits.

Sitting your backside in a tub of warm salt water is called a sitz bath, and it can alleviate some discomforts of hemorrhoids and increase circulation down there. Witch hazel and Epsom salt compresses can ease the swelling, and ice packs can help with the pain. You may want to try sleeping with your hips and legs elevated to reduce the pressure in that area. If constipation is a problem, ask your health-care provider to recommend a stool softener or topical ointment that might help. Finally, when trying to have a bowel movement, place your feet on a stool 10 to 12 inches high, take two deep cleansing breaths and exhale as you push. This should help you avoid straining, which can cause the veins in the area to swell.

Supine Hypotensive Syndrome

If you're experiencing weakness, lightheadedness, nausea and dizziness, don't overreact: it might have more to do with your posture and body position than anything more serious. When you lie on your back during the later stages of pregnancy, the blood flow from your heart may be blocked to some degree because your uterus is tilting back and pressing against your main arteries. This can cause a decrease in your heart rate and lower your blood pressure, making you feel lightheaded, nauseous and weak. This condition is called supine hypotensive syndrome, and the symptoms can be relieved simply by changing position. Instead of lying on your back, try lying on your left side. Placing a wedge under the right hip has also been observed to relieve the obstruction of blood flow. If you feel you must lie on your back, keep your upper body semi-upright, preferably at a 45-degree angle, by propping yourself against some pillows. Ultimately this condition will probably resolve itself; as your baby grows, she will start to fit herself more snugly into your pelvic area, thereby limiting the mobility of your uterus.

Insomnia

Do you remember when you could go into your bedroom, sit on your bed and before your head hit the pillow you were asleep. And now, it's not only hard to fall asleep, but it's hard to stay asleep when you are able to get some shut-eye. Don't fret too much; insomnia is rather common in pregnancy. Most women report some level of insomnia while pregnant. The good news is the lack of sleep doesn't hurt the baby. And although it's painstaking lying in bed worrying over how little sleep you are getting, the truth is you are probably getting more sleep than you realize.

If a trip to the bathroom is all it takes to keep you up, then concentrate your fluid intake during the daytime. The temperature of your bedroom can also contribute to insomnia. Ensure that your room temperature is just right for you, not too warm and not too cold. Create a bedtime routine and try to stick to it. Start with aromatherapy. You can light incense or spritz a scent known to create restfulness like lavender, jasmine or ylang-ylang. Have a cup of chamomile tea followed by a warm shower. Be strong and leave the small screen as well as the big screen off and opt to do some reading. Our fingers are crossed for sweet dreams.

Your Baby at Seven Months

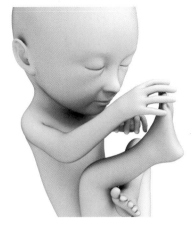

During the last three months of your pregnancy, your baby will be busy gaining most of her birth weight—probably more than a pound this month alone. If born prematurely, a fetus at this age has a good chance of survival. Although she may not yet be able to keep herself adequately warm due to the lack of fat under her skin, her lungs are now capable of breathing air. Her nervous system has also matured enough to direct rhythmic breathing motions. Neonatal intensive care units are equipped with the technology to compensate for a baby's inability to control her body temperature, but of course there are various other dangers associated with being born this early. The baby may have difficulty breathing and her digestive tract may not function adequately. The premature baby is also vulnerable to infections. But medical professionals work hard to protect and care for preemies until they are strong enough to thrive on their own.

While still in your womb, your baby may begin to practice her sucking skills. She will also start yawning, swallowing and making breathing movements, all in preparation for her life on the outside. The hair on her head may grow longer, and she may shed lanugo, the downy hair covering her body. As the lanugo fades away, the greasy coating of vernix caseosa thickens.

As her kidneys begin to mature, she will start to pass urine, and the vernix provides a layer of protection so her skin won't get irritated. The fact that babies are swallowing their amniotic fluid at this point—and therefore their own urine—isn't as gross as it sounds. It's all really just the same fluid in and out. The vernix will be helpful during her journey through the birth canal as well. A greased-up, lubricated baby is definitely easier to push through the 10 centimeters of space your body provides. Trust us; you'll be happy for all of the help you can get to ensure that your labor and delivery are as easy and safe as possible.

Your baby's eyelids are no longer fused; she can now blink and react to light. She might even move around a bit if you shine a bright light on your abdomen, as unborn babies are known to turn toward bright lights.

Prenatal Care at Seven Months

At this point, you will probably start visiting your health-care provider every 2 weeks instead of once a month. During this month's visits, your provider will probably want to give you the tetanus, diphtheria and pertussis vaccine, better known as the Tdap vaccine. Whether you've received this vaccination prior or not, the Centers for Disease Control and Prevention recommends that it be given at each pregnancy.

Tdap is a combination vaccination that protects pregnant women against three potentially life-threatening bacterial diseases: tetanus, diphtheria and pertussis. If acquired through a cut or a wound, tetanus can affect the brain and the nervous system. Diphtheria is contagious and makes it difficult to breathe and pertussis is whooping cough, an extremely contagious respiratory infection. It's important to give this vaccination to pregnant women because it is expected to pass through the placenta and likely provide some protection to their babies. These are the very good reasons your provider would want to administer the Tdap vaccine. The most optimal time for administering Tdap during pregnancy is between your seventh and ninth months. Tdap is routinely given and is not known to elevate the frequency of adverse events in pregnancy.

The GCT is also routinely given during pregnancy around your seventh month. This test screens for gestational diabetes as it measures your response to sugar. Gestational diabetes is a condition that affects pregnant women who have never had diabetes before but who now have high glucose or sugar levels. There is a full description of gestational diabetes in Chapter 3. The GCT does not diagnose gestational diabetes, so a positive result doesn't mean you have gestational diabetes. The test identifies who may be at risk for it, thereby needing the full three-hour Gestational tolerance test.

As usual, your provider will also want to check the following this month:

- Your weight
- Your blood pressure
- Your fundal height
- The fetal heartbeat
- Your hands and feet for swelling, and your legs for varicose veins
- Your uterine size and the growth of your baby (through abdominal palpation and measurement)
- Any unusual symptoms

If your health-care provider has determined that you are at high risk for any disorder that can affect your baby's growth, including hypertension or diabetes, for example, ultrasound surveillance will begin this month. This ongoing observation will give your provider the information she or he needs to make critical decisions that will keep both you and your baby healthy and safe for the duration of your pregnancy and childbirth.

Don't forget your list of questions and concerns!

Writing a Birth Plan

You've probably been doing some thinking about the kind of childbirth experience you would like to have. If you haven't, you should revisit Chapter 9 to review the childbirth options available for you and your family. Now may be a good time for you and your partner to give some serious thought to how you would like your labor and childbirth scenario to play out, and then write down a birth plan. This birth plan poses a wonderful opportunity for you as a couple to actually visualize the scene of you bringing forth your child into the world.

Your plan, for example, can include the option of receiving an epidural under certain conditions. If you'd prefer to have your own pillow or wear your own gown, rather than one supplied by the hospital, include that in your plan as well. You might have opinions about the ambiance of your birthing room. Would you prefer dimmed lights? Is there any particular background music you'd like to be playing during your labor? These things can be part of your plan, too. Any reasonable and safe personal preference can certainly be put on the table, though some may not be feasible.

Whether or not you put it down on paper, you actually started creating your birth plan way back during your first few weeks of pregnancy, when you began interviewing health-care providers. If you asked the right questions then, and found the right professional partner, your vision and objectives for your labor and delivery shouldn't be a surprise or a problem for your health-care provider. Giving birth is a collaborative effort between a family and a medical team, and it's important to have consensus on the issues that are important to you.

Here are some more issues that you might want to address in your plan:

- The degree to which your partner will be involved in the labor and birth (of course you'll want to discuss this between yourselves)
- Whether or not you'd like the option of eating or drinking during labor
- Whether or not you'd like your pubic hair shaved
- How you feel about the use of enemas or suppositories
- How you feel about fetal monitoring procedures
- Whether you'd like to be able to move around freely during various stages of labor
- The amount and kind of pain relief you might want during labor
- How strongly you feel about spontaneous versus medically induced labor
- Your feelings about an episiotomy, do you want it only if absolutely necessary (We fully explain this and many of the other procedures listed here in Chapter 14)
- Whether you'd like to be able to touch your baby's head during crowning
- Whether your partner wants to be the one to cut the umbilical cord

Here is just one example of a birth plan. The format and the content can be as unique as you are. You can write your plan as a letter or just list all of your preferences, and what you include in your plan is up to you. Once you are happy with all of the details, deliver the plan to your health-care provider and be ready to discuss it at your next visit.

Sample Birth Plan

Thank you for all of the valuable information about pregnancy, labor and childbirth. It has helped me tremendously. With all of this knowledge, I am aware that there are many things that I can do to make my childbirth experience smooth and fulfilling. Ámon and I have thought carefully about how we would like the birth of our child to be and have included our preferences in the following plan:

- We'd like to remain at home for as long as it is safely possible.
- Once at the hospital, we'd like to be allowed free mobility during labor, with intermittent monitoring of the baby.
- I'd like to be allowed to eat light snacks or drink juices during early labor.
- I'd prefer not to have my pubic area shaved.
- I'd like to avoid suppositories if possible but am willing to use them if necessary.
- I would like to wear my own T-shirt, rather than a hospital gown, during delivery.
- I would like my amniotic sac to be allowed to break spontaneously.
- I would prefer to deliver the baby in a squatting or semi-upright position, if possible.
- If it is clear that I will need pain medication to proceed with a vaginal delivery, I would prefer an epidural or spinal so that I can move around and remain aware of my contractions.
- I'd like to avoid an episiotomy, if possible.
- I intend to breast-feed and would like to do it as soon as the baby is born.

I am truly looking forward to this extraordinary experience in my life. Thank you again.

Your Pregnancy & Your Man

Our "Your Pregnancy & Your Man" feature wouldn't be legit if we didn't take time to focus on a key concern for men faced with impending parenthood: money!

Men bring their emotions to every aspect of the pregnancy experience, and the issue of money is no exception. For that reason, it is crucial to be a good listener. Try to understand his financial concerns and take them seriously. Don't try to make a dollar out of fifteen cents, the way we sometimes do. Financial planning is a process, and the first step in that process is listening. Once your man feels his concerns have been heard and that you are in the financial struggle together, you can move on to the number crunching, budgeting and priority setting.

Wisdom from Our Ancestors
TRADITIONAL LABOR & BIRTH

Now that you are thinking seriously about your own labor and birth, it's a good time to take a look at how our ancestors managed this special time.

One thing is clear: priority was given to creating a birth situation that was most relaxing for the mother. This often included having a network of family members present, thus creating a very warm and joyous mood. The birthing event resembled a family social gathering in celebration of the laboring woman.

Since there was no such thing as an episiotomy, traditional women often steamed, oiled and massaged the perineum (*per-eh-NEE-ehm*), the area between the vagina and the anus, so that it could stretch and allow the infant to pass. It was important that the perineum be made flexible so as to avoid tearing. Women steamed their genital areas by squatting over a pot of herbs on a fire in order to thin the tissue and make it suppler. They also sat in shallow baths of herbal preparations during the last few weeks of pregnancy to relax this special tissue. Lubricating the perineum was done right before birth to relax the skin and prevent it from splitting, especially if the birth attendant feared that the birth would be dry. A labor and birth with a low amount of amniotic fluid can be called a dry birth. There are a number of reasons why amniotic fluid can be low. Babies who remain in the womb too long can start to produce less amniotic fluid. Low fluid levels are also caused by too much fluid leaking out prior to active labor.

During labor, women often sat astride a hammock or squatted close to the ground, also to help prevent tearing. To avoid the baby's head from pushing out too abruptly, soft counterpressure could be applied using the hammock or a pile of cloths or skins. This helped ease the baby's head out slowly, allowing time for the perineum to expand and give way without damage. And even if some tearing did occur, the tears were minimal and would heal well, especially with the help of folk remedies used by many African tribes.

To Do This Month

A Quick Checklist

☐ Buy a well-fitting nursing bra if milk begins to leak from your nipples.

☐ Buy nursing pads.

☐ Be mindful of your posture to avoid slouching and ultimately backache.

☐ Rest when you need it.

☐ Go to the bathroom whenever you feel the urge—never hold it in.

☐ Lie on your left side whenever possible.

☐ Start writing out your birth plan with your partner.

☐ Listen to your man's thoughts about the finances.

☐ Make a copy of the Prenatal Appointment Schedule Worksheet (page 210) and jot down your questions.

☐ Go to this month's prenatal care appointments.

☐ Get your Tdap vaccine from your provider.

☐ Take the GCT from your provider.

CHAPTER 12

The Eighth Month
Weeks 31-35

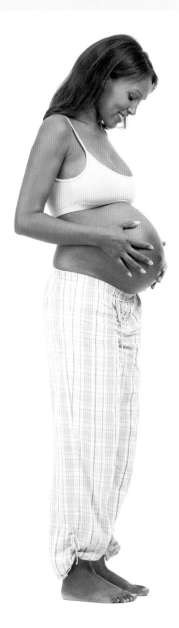

Your body is now hard at work preparing you for labor. You may be feeling uncomfortable, but you have to admit how remarkable and capable your body is as it makes all sorts of adjustments to bring forth new life.

How You Look

One thing that has certainly changed now is the way you walk. Because of your big, beautiful belly, your center of gravity has shifted. To compensate for the extra weight pulling you forward, you are probably arching your back to keep your balance. This can lead to the typical waddling walk pregnant women are known for. Safety while walking is very important, so watch out for cracks, ditches, steps and other obstacles. Wear low-heeled shoes and consider a maternity girdle or maternity belt for stability and relief of lower back pain. You can buy these at most maternity clothing stores. Another reason to remain vigilant as you move around is because you may find yourself daydreaming more and generally feeling less focused. Call it "the pregnancy haze." Some of us believe that the "haze" never really clears up, since from pregnancy we go straight into sleep deprivation that comes with caring for a newborn. It's all good, though. That sweet-smelling bundle of joy won't mind; he loves you, haze and all. Plus when it comes right down to it, you'll always be there 100 percent for him.

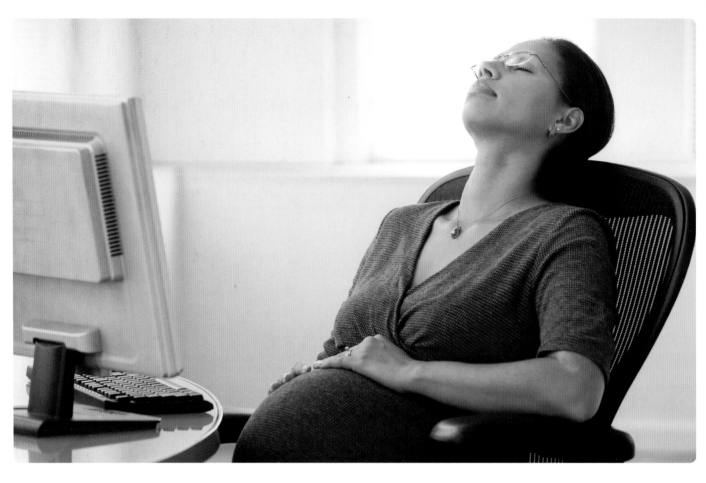

How You May Feel

Let's just state the obvious: you are a lot bigger now, so everything you feel is more intense, from back aches to hunger to your constant need to urinate. You're just 8 weeks from the extraordinary experience of childbirth, and some discomfort comes with the territory.

Braxton-Hicks Contractions

At this point, you might begin to feel Braxton-Hicks contractions. These rhythmic constrictions of the uterus can take the form of a tightening or pulling sensation in the upper belly area, pulling in the thighs, downward pressure in the pelvic area or backache. Please understand that these are quite normal; think of them as your uterus exercising in preparation for labor and birth. They have nothing to do with your cervix opening or expanding, as it will on the big day. When Braxton-Hicks contractions do occur, you can try the breathing exercises you've been learning in childbirth class. These should relax you, and the practice is beneficial, too. If you're doing something active when you feel a contraction, stop, rest and massage your stomach lightly.

Backache

When you think about what you are now carrying around and the stress it causes to the ligaments and muscles of your lower back and spine, it's no surprise that you are experiencing back pain. (In fact, it would be a surprise if you weren't.) This pain is quite normal, but you can ameliorate the discomfort by adopting a "tall" posture when sitting or standing. Tilt your pelvis forward and keep your buttocks tucked under as much as possible. Try to avoid any heavy lifting—and that includes your children—but if you must lift something or someone, squat down with your knees bent to do it, rather than bending over at the waist. And when explaining your behavior to your kids, don't blame the baby for your moratorium on picking them up. You don't want big brother or sister feeling anything but excitement about their new sibling!

A firm mattress or a bed board under the mattress can provide extra support for your back during these last few months. Try sleeping on your side with your upper leg supported on pillows. Back massages are very beneficial now, too, and they don't have to be professional ones. See Chapter 4 for some good massage techniques your partner can learn.

If your upper back is aching, it may be due to an increase in the size of your breasts. (They might be a bit tender as well. It all comes with the territory.) There are no miracle cures for the aches and pains you are feeling now, but knowing that your discomfort is normal and that it will go away after birth should help you relax and cope with it. Meanwhile, wear well-fitted bras, maintain good posture (shoulders back) and stretch your arms over your head frequently to exercise the muscles of your upper back.

Itchy Skin

The mild itching you may be experiencing is primarily due to the increased blood flow to your skin. Abdominal itching may also be due to the stretching of your skin to cover that beautiful, blossoming belly. Try moisturizing regularly to relieve the surface tension and wear loose-fitting clothing to eliminate the extra irritation that rubbing can cause. A breathable fabric such as 100 percent cotton is your best bet, as it will allow air to circulate over the surface of your skin. Cool baths can be soothing as well, followed by a generous amount of moisturizer to replenish essential oils.

Leg Cramps

You may be feeling some leg cramps or shooting pains in your thighs and buttocks. These are probably caused by the pressure your uterus is putting on nerves and blood vessels, thus impairing circulation to your legs. Exercise can ease this discomfort. Elevate your legs periodically throughout the day and avoid lying on your stomach with your toes pointed.

Cramps can also be caused by an imbalance of calcium, phosphorus and magnesium in your body, so consult with your health-care provider if the cramps are persistent. She or he may recommend increasing the amount of calcium in your diet, which you can do by drinking a couple of extra glasses of milk each day. If you're lactose intolerant, try foods rich in calcium such as salmon and dark leafy vegetables.

Varicose Veins

In addition to leg cramps, women in the latter stages of pregnancy are prone to varicose veins—those weird, red and blue squiggly lines that can run along your calf and up your leg. These veins are responsible for returning blood to your heart, and they look like that when they swell up from working hard to move your blood upward against gravity. Again, your enlarged uterus may be a contributing factor, as it compresses your veins and compromises your circulation.

There's often a genetic component to varicose veins, so you might want to find out if they run in your family. They can be sore to the touch and itchy, and they can make your legs feel tired or heavy. Support socks won't prevent varicose veins but they can help alleviate the discomfort. Avoid crossing your legs (that is, if you still can with that belly of yours). Elevate your legs whenever you can and try lying on your left side. All of these things should help your circulation. And keep in mind that your varicose veins will become much less visible—if not disappear completely—after childbirth.

Discharge

Vaginal discharge may increase now due to the increase in blood flow to your cervix and the mucus that forms because of your increased level of estrogen. Your vaginal secretions have become more acidic as part of your body's natural drive to control the bacteria that can cause infection. Infection control, especially in this area, is of utmost importance now—so be proud that your body is taking care of business.

Numbness

During the last couple of months of your pregnancy, you may experience numbness and tingling of your fingers and toes. There are a few theories as to why this is. It has been suggested that an enlarged uterus pressing on the veins and nerves that supply the legs and toes can cause numbness. Swelling may also cause pressure and tingling of hands and feet, especially upon rising in the morning. The swelling of tissue associated with carpal tunnel syndrome (a painful disorder of the wrist and hands) has been identified as a possible cause of numbness of the arm. Vitamin B deficiency has also been cited as a cause of numbness, as has decreased carbon dioxide from hyperventilation.

There are as many suggestions for relief or management of numbness and tingling as there are theories for its existence. Since swelling has been identified as a culprit, following the suggestions for relief of swelling in Chapter 10 may help. Remove rings and constricting jewelry, and exercise your hands periodically. Make sure you are eating well and that your diet is well balanced. You might want to wear a wrist splint while sleeping to help reduce pain in the hands, wrists and arms. If you remain bothered by numbness and tingling, call your health-care provider, who may be able to suggest additional remedies. But the fact is that numbness and tingling of the fingers and toes may be one of the discomforts of pregnancy that simply has to be tolerated.

Your Baby at Eight Months

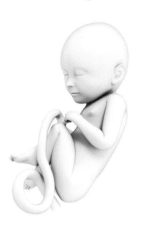

By the eighth month of gestation, your unborn baby will weigh about 4 pounds and measure about 12 inches from head to rump. He has gained these extra pounds mostly in a protective layer of fat under his skin, which will keep his body warm after birth. All of the changes he experiences now are the result of his body preparing him for life outside of the womb. His legs and arms have grown chubby and his skin has smoothed out. His brain and nerves are maturing and will continue to do so until birth and beyond.

He now fits so snugly within your womb that he is no longer able to practice gymnastics but can only move a little from side to side. Very soon he will probably assume a head-down position. Most babies do, because the head is their heaviest and largest body part, and it is best accommodated in the bottom contour of the uterus.

Your baby can now hear the many sounds of his world, most notably your stomach rumblings, your heartbeat and your voice. Because these sounds will be quite familiar to him by the time he is born, placing him on your chest immediately after birth may be very calming as he confronts the bright, noisy and totally unfamiliar world of the delivery room.

Throughout month 8, your baby will continue to practice his breathing movements in preparation for his first gulp of air. This rhythmic movement of his diaphragm and chest wall is vital to helping his lungs mature.

Prenatal Care at Eight Months

At this month's visits with your health-care provider, he or she will probably check the following:

- Your weight
- Your blood pressure
- Your fundal height
- The fetal heartbeat
- Your urine for sugar and protein
- Your hands and feet for swelling, and your legs for varicose veins
- Your uterine size and the growth of your baby (through abdominal palpation and measurement)
- Any unusual symptoms

Don't forget your list of questions and concerns, which at this point may include issues related to the childbirth experience itself.

Now that you've reached 32 weeks, your health-care provider will probably want to take another good look at your baby, so an ultrasound may be performed. This will be used to check your baby's presentation, or which part of him is facing down. Don't be alarmed if his head isn't occupying the lower portion of your uterus yet; not all babies are head down at 32 weeks. By 35 weeks, though, his head should be nestled into the contours of your pelvis. (You'll find more about your baby's presentation in Chapter 13.)

The ultrasound will also be used to assess your baby's weight, height, the growth of his body parts and the amount of amniotic fluid you are producing. Your doctor really just wants to make sure that your baby is developing as expected.

Your Pregnancy & Your Man

It's pretty obvious that you and your mate are in transition. It's a changeover from being a couple to being a family, and it affects every couple differently. But one thing is certain: the quality of your relationship forms the emotional climate into which your baby is born. That may seem obvious, but it's important to think about. Your child's emotional stability matters right from birth and is as important to his growth as the state of his bones and muscles. A child subjected to fear or emotional pain is facing obstacles to his social and even intellectual development.

So what if the quality of your relationship is a little shaky? The Alliance for Early Success's Birth through Age Eight State Policy Framework identified family stress as a factor that can compromise the parent-child relationship, thereby limiting precious opportunities for stimulating and responsive interactions, emotional support and activities that enrich children's health, knowledge and skills. Now that you know how profound the impact of your own relationship can be on your child, it's up to both you and your mate to do something about it. Your pregnancy comes with a commitment on both of your parts to being loving, supportive people—to each other and to your newborn.

As you are well aware, children require a great deal of care in many forms, but love is probably the most important of them all. Make sure you provide your baby with a loving and nurturing environment, and carefully monitor the relationships and behaviors he is exposed to. This is your best bet in providing him with a foundation for strong emotional health.

Wisdom from Our Ancestors
BLACK FOLK MYTHS & SUPERSTITIONS
LABOR & CHILDBIRTH

You're scrubbing every floor in the house, including the carpets. You're painting rooms and cooking meals that'll last a week. It can only mean one thing: you're going into labor soon. Is this a sign or just good planning? Either way, as the big day approaches, the folk wisdom flies thick and fast. Here are some other superstitions about the final phases of the birth process that you may want to take with a few grains of salt:

- When your naval drops, you're ready to deliver.
- Sitting in a tub of hot water will jump-start your labor.
  Reality Check: Beware of sitting in water that's too hot, such as in a hot tub. This can raise your temperature to a dangerous level.
- Rubbing your stomach daily with dirty dishwashing water will ensure an easy delivery.
- To ensure a healthy delivery, don't let anyone sweep under the bed where the birth will take place.
  Reality Check: On the other hand, a clean and sanitary environment is good for everyone!
- Burn or bury your afterbirth to keep from hemorrhaging or experiencing other complications.
- Mix cobwebs and soot with sugar, then place the concoction in the vaginal tract to prevent postnatal hemorrhaging.
  Reality Check: You know what we're going to say: please don't put anything into your vaginal tract! You'll be setting the stage for a mega-infection if you do.

To Do This Month

A Quick Checklist

- ☐ Get a maternity girdle and wear low-heeled shoes for stability and lower-back pain relief, if needed.

- ☐ Keep a "tall" posture when sitting or standing.

- ☐ Avoid heavy lifting.

- ☐ Elevate your legs periodically throughout the day.

- ☐ Strengthen your loving relationships.

- ☐ Make a copy of the Prenatal Appointment Schedule Worksheet (page 210) and jot down your questions.

- ☐ Go to this month's prenatal care appointments.

CHAPTER 13

The Ninth Month

Weeks 36-40

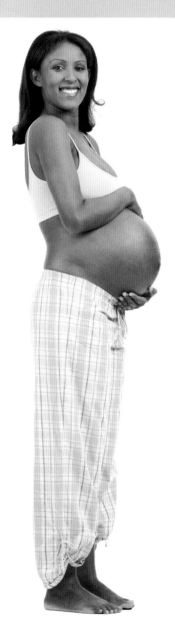

Well, this is it! This is the last month you will have to tolerate the rather extreme body changes and discomforts of pregnancy. But more important than anything else is that you get your life's gift! You will finally get to meet your baby. You'll get to hold the little one who took up residence in the safe and nurturing environment of your womb.

How You Look

You're looking great. This is the time when pregnancy is truly an awesome phenomenon. Your body has stretched itself to the fullest to accommodate another human being, and most of us marvel at such a beautiful sight. You may not be able to appreciate it because you're being pushed to the limits, but you really are astonishing to others. This process is a special miracle.

How You May Feel

You have about 4 more weeks until your body will begin the journey of feeling like *your* body again. Until then, you'll have to endure a bit more discomfort.

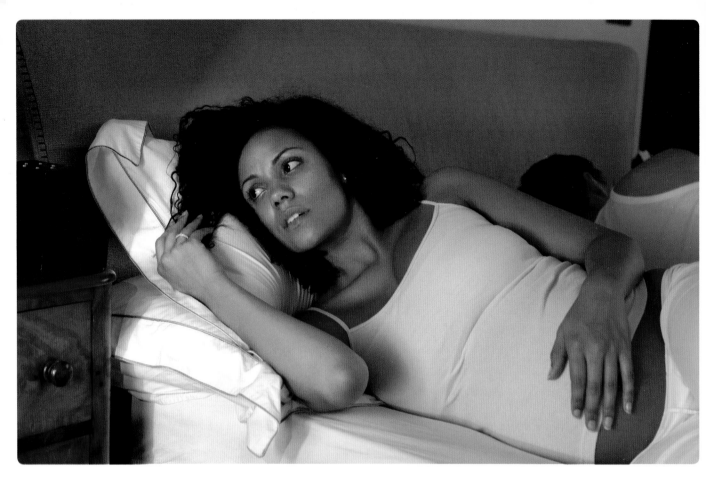

Pubic Area Pain

At this point you can expect to have some pain around your pubic area. Since your pubic tissues are beginning to stretch, your pelvic joints are becoming more relaxed and excessively mobile. This is natural and necessary; ultimately, it will enable your body to pass a 6- to 9-pound, 17-inch baby through your pelvic cavity, but right now this change may be causing painful strain to your muscles and ligaments. Consider wearing a girdle or maternity corset that will decrease movement and provide much-needed support. Maintaining correct posture will also reduce excess strain on pelvic joints.

Lightening

If it hasn't already, lightening will occur during your ninth month. It's when your baby's head (or rump if she is in a breech position), slips deep into your pelvic cavity. When this happens, you will probably be able to breathe more easily, since she is no longer pushing against your diaphragm.

Sleeping Challenges

Sleeping and resting may be more difficult now due to your large belly, which makes finding a comfortable position seem nearly impossible. We encourage you to rest whenever you feel tired since labor is approaching, and you will be better able to meet its demands if you are rested rather than exhausted.

Producing Milk

Just as the sounds of your heartbeat and voice calm and nurture your baby's emotional needs, your body will produce colostrum, or "first milk," to fulfill her physical needs. You are truly your baby's life support, and colostrum is what you produce before your true milk comes in. Toward the end of your pregnancy, you may notice your nipples discharging this light, thin and milky substance, which is filled with antibodies and other immune-boosting substances. If you choose to breast-feed, your baby will be the beneficiary of this natural protection—but for now you may need to put breast pads into your bra to prevent staining and wet spots on your clothing. There is nothing stranger-looking than two big wet spots on a pretty blouse.

Burst of Energy

Surprisingly, at this point in your pregnancy you may experience a burst of energy, driving you to clean, wash, cook and even paint. It's all part of the nesting instinct, so go ahead and take advantage of it, but don't overdo it. Remember that the job ahead of you will require all of the energy you can summon up. Get those chores done but rest as much as you can between washing and folding your newborn's clothing and rearranging that nursery for the tenth time.

Your Baby at Nine Months

Your baby is quite plump now, though her growth has slowed down considerably. By the end of this month, babies may weigh anywhere from 6 to 9 pounds and measure on average 17 inches from head to toe. Most of the lanugo (fine downy hair) has fallen off, and you may see some remnants of vernix (greasy, cheese-like substance) after birth in her body creases, around her neck and in the folds of her skin. Her nails have probably grown past her fingertips, which is why she may be born with scratches on her face. You will probably have to trim them soon after birth. As her head slips into the tight circle of your pelvic bones (lightening), she will most likely be pinned down with her face toward your back. She is now ready for her trip through the birth canal. But even in those tight quarters, she will continue kicking, stretching and squirming. If you ever go too long without feeling her move, call your health-care provider immediately.

Prenatal Care at Nine Months

From here on in, you will probably have to visit your doctor or midwife once a week. At these visits, your health-care provider will probably check the following:

- Your weight
- Your blood pressure
- Your fundal height
- The fetal heartbeat
- Your urine for sugar and protein
- Group B streptococcus culture (GBS) is taken in the last trimester of pregnancy to identify the presence of harmful bacteria that could be passed on to the baby during labor and delivery.
- Blood count
- HIV testing
- Your hands and feet for swelling, and your legs for varicose veins
- Your uterine size and the growth of your baby (through abdominal palpation and measurement)
- Engagement and presentation of baby

As far as your baby's position is concerned, now is when it's crucial. Her head should be nestled in the circle of your pelvic bones. If she is not presenting head down but rather in a breech position, your health-care provider may suggest turning her manually, which is called version. This procedure involves attempting to move the baby into a head-down position by manipulating her from the outside of your belly. It is conducted with the help of sonography in the hospital or your provider's medical office. If you chose not to undergo this process, your options include cesarean section or a vaginal breech birth. These are very important decisions and should be made by you and your provider together after a thorough discussion of the pros and cons. Good luck!

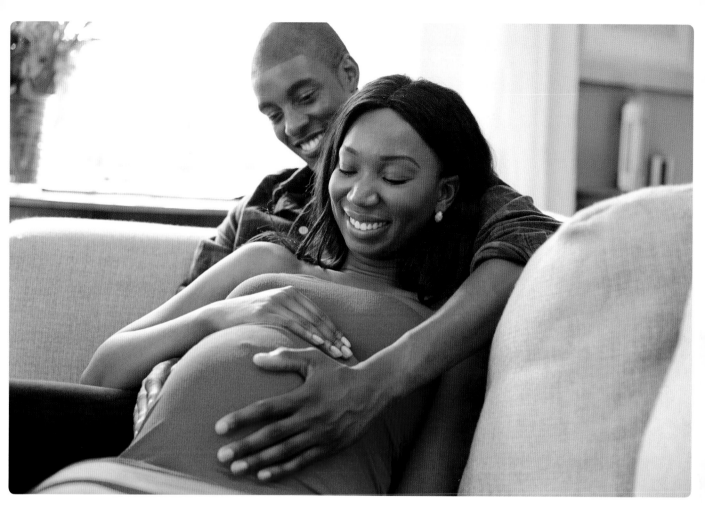

Your Pregnancy & Your Man

As the actual labor and delivery date approaches, your man will probably become more concerned about your health. He'll be thinking about the pain you will go through and may fear his own inability to help you through it. Although some men wouldn't miss the experience for the world, many are ambivalent about being in the delivery room for the birth. Some clearly aren't ambivalent at all and would rather be almost anywhere else. At the end of the day, he knows how much his presence means to you and will probably overcome his own fear to be at your side.

The decision to be present during childbirth is personal, though, so keep in mind that a father's absence shouldn't compromise his relationship with his child—or you.

Wisdom from Our Ancestors
A FLASHBACK IN TIME

Just about nowhere in the tribal world did women lie down once labor began and not get up until the birth was over. Remaining inactive is a very modern method of doing things. Quite conversely, many tribal women purposely engaged in physical activity in order to bring on labor and birth. Rather than assuming a passive role, they took the whole process into their own hands. On a deep, instinctive level—and with the help and coaching of their mothers and female elders—they understood their bodies and the birth process and how to get through it successfully.

Walking was one of the more common ways women accelerated their labor, although lifting moderately heavy objects at a critical time during labor was also done to increase the intensity of the contractions and bring on birth.

Birth attendants were usually present to provide the mother with physical support, and that included massage. Across just about all traditional societies, massage has been used during childbirth, generally focused on the back and thighs as well as on the upper part of the mother's abdomen. Massage was also used to reposition babies who were breech or in some other unsafe position for delivery.

The use of massage wasn't limited to just labor and birth. In fact, women were massaged throughout their pregnancies, primarily to improve their muscle tone and physical endurance during labor and birth. Massage might also be employed during the new mother's recovery period to help rejuvenate the uterus and revive menstrual flow.

Now you know what some of our great-great-grandmothers did during pregnancy and childbirth. It's safe to say that they put the *natural* in natural childbirth. Although we are fortunate to have doctors, midwives, hospitals and equipment at our disposal, we think it pays to draw wisdom and strength from our elders' example. After all, we're here because of them.

To Do This Month

A Quick Checklist

- ☐ Rest whenever you feel tired, if you can.

- ☐ Use breast pads to prevent staining cloths, if you leak.

- ☐ Make a copy of the Prenatal Appointment Schedule Worksheet (page 210) and jot down your questions.

- ☐ Go to this month's prenatal care appointments.

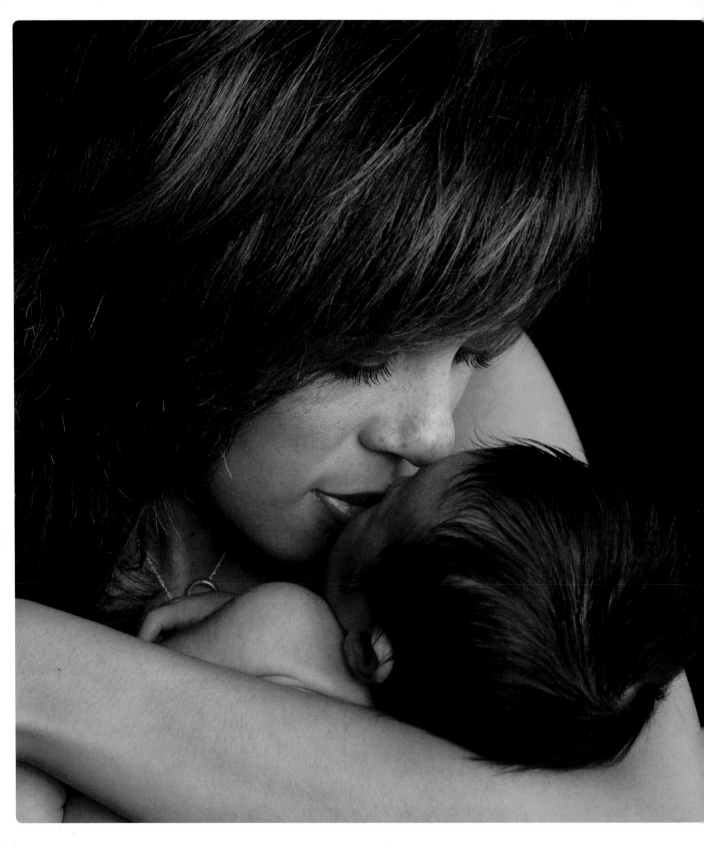

PART III

The World Has One More Chance for Improvement: A Beautiful Black Baby Is Born!

And born your child will be, into greatness and beauty with unlimited potential. But before you can celebrate this blessed event, you are going to have to work for it; that's why it's called *labor*.

No one ever said giving birth was easy, but one of the miraculous things about it is that once it's over, the pain is forgotten while the joy remains. Otherwise, who would choose to do it all over again? So, while you may be cringing at the thought of a 7-pound baby squeezing through your birth canal and, well, you know the story, there's something about the process of bringing forth new life that makes all of the physical changes, the aches and pains, and even that big final effort worthwhile. And isn't it remarkable how our bodies know just what to do at the right time? Bones that have never moved or expanded for any other reason widen during childbirth in order to accommodate a baby's head. What an extraordinary body we possess.

It might comfort you to think of your pain as your badge of honor for bringing life into the world. And once your child is here, a celebration is indeed called for.

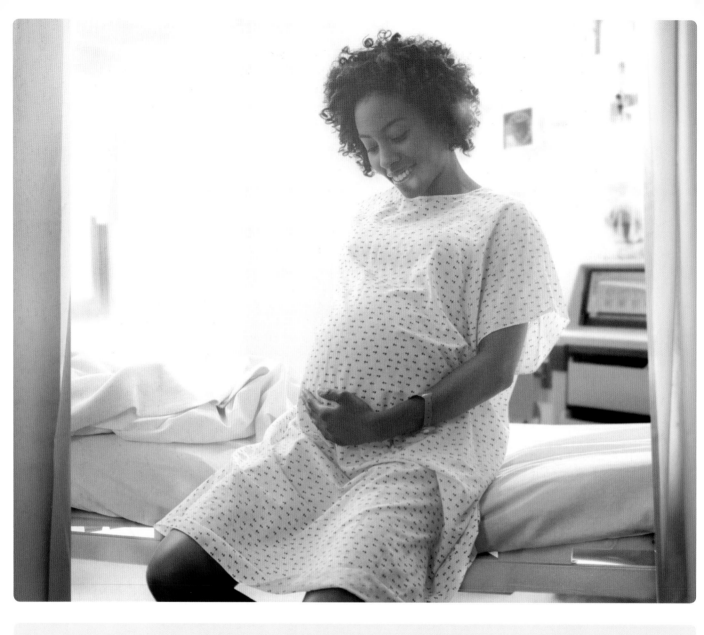

CHAPTER 14

Labor & Delivery

After all of those weeks of waiting, the grand finale is finally here. With it comes feelings of excitement as well as concern as you begin to anticipate the act of labor and the prospect of seeing your baby for the first time. A few nerves are understandable, but it's important to avoid letting them get the best of you. The more knowledgeable you are about what happens to your body and your baby during labor and birth, the less anxious you will be.

We feel it's important for you to understand the process from start to finish so you can prepare for it mentally as well as physically. The first thing to understand is that there is no wrong or right labor and delivery. Every woman experiences the process in a unique way and even the same woman will have different experiences for different births.

Your Body, Your Baby, Your Choice

If you are planning on a hospital delivery, it comes with its own protocols. Hospitals are institutions, of course, dedicated primarily to healing people who are sick and injured. The good people who work in them navigate life-or-death situations every day, so adherence to strict policies and procedures is necessary. As a laboring woman in a hospital setting, you are a bit of an outlier. Assuming your pregnancy has been healthy and low-risk, you are neither sick nor injured and you require minimal intervention, since nature has provided you with everything you need to bring life into the world. It can be a challenge to stick to the birth plan you've decided on as you are faced with diligent staff members eager to abide by hospital policies. You may find yourself subjected to a variety of routine of tests and monitoring methods that you don't understand—and perhaps don't need or want.

This doesn't mean you should rule out a hospital delivery; just that if you want to be a decision maker throughout the process, you must remain vigilant in communicating your wishes to your caregivers and insisting that they consult you fully on all procedures. This is easier if you've developed a birth plan ahead of time. (See Chapter 11 for more on that process.)

Packing Your Bag

Giving birth would be a whole lot easier if you knew exactly when it was going to happen, but there is usually an element of surprise surrounding a baby's actual birthday. For that reason, you should have your bags packed at least two weeks prior to your due date. Here are some of the things you should consider taking with you to the hospital or birth center:

FOR YOU

- A cotton nightgown or T-shirt to wear during labor. You may feel more comfortable in your own clothing rather than in a hospital gown.
- A couple of nightgowns for after the birth. Make sure they button down the front if you plan to nurse.
- A few pairs of panties and some bras. Make them nursing bras if you're going to breast-feed and include nursing pads.
- Your bathrobe.
- Nonslip slippers.
- Your toiletries (toothbrush, toothpaste, deodorant, soap, lip balm, sanitary pads—not tampons—and all of the little extras [moisturizers, mouthwash, etc.] that make you feel good).
- Thick socks, as your feet might get cold during labor.
- Cosmetics.
- Eyeglasses or extra contact lenses and solutions.
- Your favorite pillow, since hospital pillows tend to be flat.
- A little bit of pocket money—but go easy on the valuables, as you don't want to have to worry about theft or loss.
- Hair accessories (hair oil, bobby pins for wrapping hair, silk scarf, headband, scrunchie—anything you need for controlling your hair during labor).
- Reading matter to entertain and distract yourself during labor. (You might even want to bring your birth announcements to work on.)
- Loose, comfortable clothing to wear home.

FOR DAD (OR OTHER LABOR COACH)

- A watch with a second hand. Timing those contractions provides valuable information about the progress of your labor.
- His favorite music and headphones.
- Oils for aromatherapy and massages.
- A video or still camera, if you've agreed to film or shoot the birth. (Make sure that you've discussed and are comfortable with the parameters here.)
- Hard candy or lollipops to keep your mouth moist.

- A washcloth to wipe your forehead.
- Snacks for both of you. (Yours might be for after the delivery.)
- Health insurance information or hospital preregistration paperwork.

FOR YOUR NEWBORN

- An undershirt or onesie.
- Diapers.
- Socks.
- Outer clothing appropriate for the season.
- Receiving blanket.
- Safety-approved car seat (it's the law in all 50 states!).

These lists make a good starting point, but think it through and add anything you feel might make all three of you happier and more comfortable during this important time.

The Progression of Labor & Delivery

There are three distinct stages in the labor and delivery process. The first stage commences when you start to experience contractions and ends when you're ready to push your baby out. This phase is all about those regular contractions and waiting for your cervix to widen. The second stage is the main event—birth—and it moves quickly and eventfully. And the third postclimactic stage comes after your baby has been born; it's when you deliver your placenta. At that point, you will probably be preoccupied with the state of your baby's health and its gender (if you don't already know it), but this is quite an important aspect of the birth process.

Let's look at each stage in turn.

Stage One: The Curtain Goes Up

You feel something. You may not know exactly what it is, but it is a new sensation, and it intensifies over time. It may be a cramp-like pain or a backache, or you may feel wetness from your broken water (amniotic sac). You'll need to determine whether you're truly in labor, and many first-time moms worry about whether they'll be able to do this. In fact, it can be a little tricky, since you may have been having those Braxton-Hicks contractions we talked about in Chapter 12. The difference is that labor contractions are more painful and occur at regular intervals. Once they begin, they'll continue more and more frequently until your baby is born. That's why it's important for you to keep track of the time between them as well as how long they last. (As you get closer to the birth, your contractions can last from 60 to 90 seconds.)

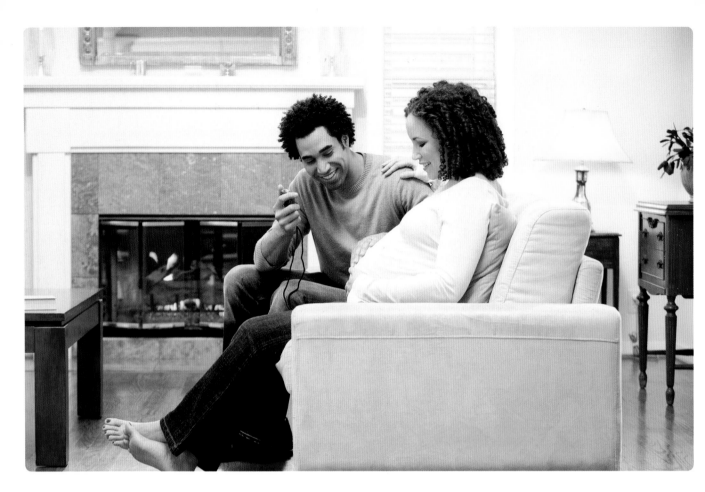

If you are feeling painful, regular contractions or there is a pinkish discharge trickling or flowing out of your vagina, you should call your doctor or midwife. She will ask you some questions so she can assess your condition and decide whether to direct you to the hospital or tell you to wait.

There really is no standard "best time" for getting there if you're not in an emergency situation. If at any point you believe you would be happier or more comfortable in the hospital, tell your health-care provider that. She or he will probably agree with you. But be aware that a hospital is never as accommodating and private as your own home, so if you don't need to be there yet, try to hold off.

AT THE HOSPITAL

Once you're at the hospital, the staff will want to make their own determination of whether you are in labor or not. In the first stage of labor, your cervix gets progressively wider (dilated) as you experience those regular uterine contractions. If a member of the hospital team determines that you aren't yet having regular contractions or dilating, you may be sent home.

Once you are admitted, this is what you'll be assessed for:

- Your progress in labor (the frequency of your contractions, how far you've dilated)
- Your physical condition (blood pressure, temperature and other vital signs)
- The condition of your baby (heart rate and positioning)
- Whether or not your amniotic sac has ruptured

An abdominal examination is the best way to assess your progress. You are no doubt familiar with these from your prenatal exams; they involve palpating your abdomen to get an idea of your baby's size and position within your uterus. The procedure also sheds some light on the frequency, duration and strength of your contractions. The attending staff will also attempt to determine the rate at which your cervix is dilating.

Cervical dilation is usually measured in centimeters (cm). A measurement of 0 centimeters means your cervix is closed; it's a natural state up until the commencement of labor. Full dilation is 10 centimeters, which is plenty of room to accommodate Junior's head. To measure how far you've dilated, a health-care professional will perform a two-finger internal exam. This may seem somewhat unscientific—and in fact, there really is no precise measurement involved—but an experienced practitioner can gather enough information this way to make decisions about your progress.

Your own physical condition is assessed more conventionally. Your blood pressure is taken and your pulse and temperature monitored. You may also be connected to an intravenous (IV) line, and there are a couple of reasons for that. Labor is physical work; you will be expending a lot of energy and perspiring. To protect you from dehydration and help maintain your endurance, the IV line may be used to replenish your fluids. Intravenous lines also come in handy for quick delivery of pain relief medication should you need or want it at any point. The line is inserted directly into a vein in your arm, and the fluid bag is attached to a rolling stand, which can be a little cumbersome to move around, but it shouldn't take away your mobility altogether.

FETAL MONITORING

Fetal monitoring, which can be external or internal, allows caregivers to track your baby's heart rate, as well as your own contractions, and identify any potential problems that might require intervention. External monitoring is done using an ultrasound transducer positioned on your belly to detect your baby's heart rate. (You probably experienced this during prenatal exams.) Internal monitoring, which is used only after your water breaks, involves placing an electrode on your little one's precious scalp for the same reason. No one doubts the benefits of electronic fetal monitoring, but it does come with one disadvantage: these monitors can prevent you from moving around. If you are lucky enough to be in a facility that uses telemetry, or "wireless" technology, you will be able to move around and walk while transmitting the vital information your caregivers require. A fetoscope (an instrument similar to a stethoscope) is another less encumbering way of checking on a baby's vitals. You might want to ask ahead of time which of these instruments is commonly used at your birthing facility.

GETTING THROUGH THE FIRST STAGE

The first stage of labor is divided into two phases: the latent phase and the active phase.

THE LATENT PHASE

The latent phase begins at the start of your contractions and ends when your cervix has dilated to about 4 cm. Your contractions during this phase will probably cause only mild pain, be brief (from 30 to 60 seconds long) and occur every 15 to 20 minutes. This phase is the longest one of the entire labor, averaging 6 to 8 hours, though it can last a day or more. You may feel nauseous and throw up or you may have diarrhea during this period, so remaining at home as long as possible will be more convenient and comfortable for you. It's perfectly fine to engage in whatever activity feels right during this period, but you may want to pamper yourself with warm showers and rest as much as you can. As we said, the decision about how long to remain at home should be made in conjunction with your health-care provider, so keep her or him posted and be candid about when you think it's time to get to that birthing center. If your latent phase lasts too long, your provider may decide to bring you into the hospital to speed up your labor.

To store up enough energy to get through labor, try eating light foods such as dry toast, soup or Jell-O, and drink plenty of liquids such as fruit juices, ginger ale and herbal tea with honey. If you're delivering in a hospital, you may be denied solid food altogether, so be prepared for that. The reason for it involves your safety (and the hospital's liability). In the event that general anesthesia is required at any point, hospitals want to avoid the possibility that you could regurgitate and then inhale any food particles.

THE ACTIVE PHASE

Once your cervix dilates to about 4 cm, you will have reached the active phase in labor. From this point on, cervical dilation should progress at its most rapid rate. This phase lasts about 4 to 7 hours and ends when you are dilated 10 cm and ready to transition to the second stage of labor—the pushing and birth stage.

Your contractions will be stronger, come more frequently (about every 3 minutes) and last longer (45 to 60 seconds). But don't worry too much about the pain; it will only be at peak intensity for about 10 seconds of each contraction—and you've been preparing for this. The best course of action is to try to concentrate on each contraction as it comes, and rest between them. Your coach should be right there with you, reassuring you and doing whatever he or she can to ease your discomfort and remind you of the big reward at the end of the line.

If the pain becomes intolerable, of course, don't hesitate to ask for pain relief medication. This is in *no way* a sign of weakness or failure. In fact, it can be the rational thing to do. Taking some pain medication early on may help you regain your coordination and composure and recover your strength so you can proceed more confidently through the second stage of labor. (We go into more specifics about methods of pain relief later in the chapter.)

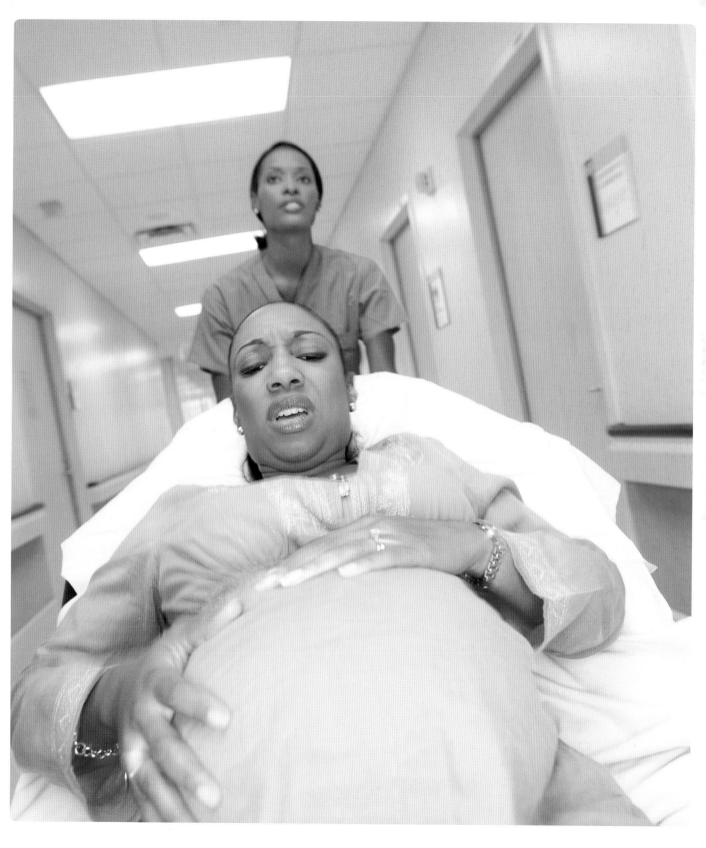

By the time you have dilated 8 to 10 cm, your body is getting ready to transition to stage two of labor. (Those last few centimeters pack a punch, and you are operating at peak energy now.) Your contractions probably feel as if they're coming right on top of each other, but they are actually about 2 to 3 minutes apart, and each one lasts about a minute. If your water hasn't broken on its own by this point, your caregiver will break it prior to the second stage of labor—but this won't hurt a bit.

The physical exertion you are experiencing now may cause your limbs to shake, and you may break into a cold sweat or feel nauseous. You may find yourself feeling irritable and discouraged. The pressure in your abdomen is probably filling you with a strong urge to push or bear down. Be prepared for the fact that if you are not yet at 10 cm, your caregivers will tell you not to do this. Listen to them! Pushing your baby's head through a cervix that's not yet wide enough to accommodate it can cause trauma to your cervix.

This is when your training is most useful. Those breathing and distraction techniques you learned in childbirth class will help you wait for the right time to push. Focus on your breathing and try changing position, which may help diminish the urge to push.

Once you've reached 10 cm, you will no longer be in the first stage of labor but will have transitioned to the second stage. This transition phase of labor can be very difficult for women because contractions are frequent, making pain intense. It may take a few minutes or up to an hour for your urge to push to kick in, which can also bring some relief from the intensity of the contractions and pain.

PAIN RELIEF

There is no standard or right way of managing pain during childbirth. Each woman's response to pain is unique and affected by a variety of factors. It's important for you to respect your own tolerance level and communicate clearly with your coach and caregivers so that together you can make the right decision about pain relief.

Understanding what your options are will help you make the right decision, too. Your experience of pain during labor and birth is affected by these factors:

- **The intensity and duration of your contractions.** The longer and more intense your contractions, the more work they accomplish in moving your baby down through your cervix. Contractions actually squeeze blood vessels that supply oxygen to your muscles. This reduction of oxygen is what causes pain.
- **The degree of your cervical dilation and the rate at which your cervix dilates with each contraction.** Shorter labors can involve more intense pain because all of the changes are occurring in a shorter amount of time. But on the other hand, the shorter your labor, the shorter the duration of the pain!

- **The stretching of the area between your vagina and rectum.** Some women eventually experience a natural anesthesia in this area because once the baby's head crowns, it can block and consequently numb the nerves in that area responsible for sending the pain message to the brain.
- **The baby's position.** Most babies position themselves with their face toward their mother's back. Some, however, are situated the other way, with the back of their head toward Mom's lower back. This can put pressure on the nerves in that area, causing what's known as back labor. In a word: ouch.

One more thing: don't underestimate the pain you can cause yourself just by thinking about the pain! The more anxious or fearful you are about what's coming, the tenser your body will be. Tense muscles can actually interfere with your contractions, which can delay labor and prolong the pain.

We know that it is hard to control your emotions, but try not to fight the pain. Rather, work on coordinating your breathing with your contractions and using your relaxation techniques. At critical moments of fear, our fight-or-flight tendencies often take over. If you are prone to the "flight" side of the equation, please plan for it going in. Talk to yourself about accepting the pain as part of the experience rather than trying to stave it off or flee from it. After all, there is nowhere to go. You are the only person who can accomplish this miracle. Women sometimes reach up and back during contractions, as if they are literally trying to get away from the pain. It's not until they pull themselves in, tuck their chins down to their chests and start to coordinate their minds with their bodies that the work gets done: the delivery of a beautiful baby boy or girl!

This is one of the reasons why childbirth education and preparation classes are so valuable. Women are taught relaxation techniques and the psychological or natural painkillers they can condition themselves to rely upon.

To manage your pain during labor and birth you can use mind-over-body strategies that don't involve pain medicine, or you can use pain-relieving drugs like anesthesia, narcotics, tranquilizers or sedatives. But just in case, here are some things you should know about both natural and synthetic pain relief.

PAIN RELIEF WITHOUT DRUGS

The most obvious solution for alleviating pain is to get away from whatever is causing it. Although that's impossible during labor, you can still plot your mental escape. Whether you believe it or not, effective use of relaxation techniques can be a natural painkiller.

First, spend some time thinking about what tends to relax you during stressful situations, so you incorporate those things into your plan. Meditation, for example, can help you focus your attention and shut out concerns, worries and pain. You can focus on a physical object such as a photo or trinket that has personal meaning, or you can focus on a word or phrase.

Music and rhythmic movement can be helpful, too. Our souls naturally respond to it, and at the right tempo and beat, it's hard not to synchronize with the rhythm. Prepare some special selections for your cell phone or portable player that can soothe and distract you. If you've listened to a particular song throughout your pregnancy, it just might soothe you (as well as your partner and your baby) during labor and birth. Or you might ask your partner to sing to you. Just think of how distracting that will be (especially if he's no Usher!).

Don't underestimate the effect of aromatherapy on the stressed-out body. Scents such as lavender, chamomile and rose are known to have calming properties. Perhaps your coach would like to incorporate these scents into your massage routine or place a few drops of them on a warm facecloth for you. Aromatherapy can help you conjure up memories or just take you to another place, either of which can help keep your mind off your pain.

Visualization involves concentrating on mental images that delight you. You might want to visualize a place where you were once happy or somewhere you'd love to be. Again, the point is to dwell on the positive rather than the pain and the discouragement that can come with it.

At this point, it might be a good idea to review the natural childbirth section in Chapter 9. There, we discuss, among other things, HypnoBirthing—a natural childbirth technique in which you use your mind to diminish pain.

The aforementioned "psychological painkillers" can all be a part of your artillery against the hard and sometimes painful work of labor and delivery, as can the following labor aides and techniques:

- Warm water or hot compresses. Take a warm shower or apply a hot compress to your back or vaginal area—or just snuggle up under a warm blanket to relieve some of your pain. Conversely, cool water or a cold compress on your face and neck can be refreshing and comforting.

- The power of touch. Being touched can create such profound effects on the human body that scientists have called it touch therapy. The slightest gesture, such as stroking a cheek or holding a hand, can convey powerful "I care and want to be with you" messages. Purposeful therapeutic massages play a big role in alleviating the pain of tense muscles. Massage can take the form of light stroking, kneading or circular pressure at strategic spots. See Chapter 4 for examples of massage techniques for the pregnant woman.

- Change positions. When you change your position during labor, your perception of pain can be diminished. Having the freedom to move into any position that makes you feel better, versus being confined, is a great start. When you change your position, you also change the relationships among gravity, your contractions, the baby and your pelvis, thus enhancing the progress of your labor. Try to remain as active as possible by doing the following:
    - Walk around.
    - Lean forward face-to-face against the person supporting you throughout your labor with your arms draped around his or her neck.

- Squat while holding onto something.
- Get on your hands and knees, especially if you are experiencing back labor.
- Sit upright in bed or on a rocking chair.

To conserve your energy and alleviate exhaustion, try alternating an active position with a resting one. If you do choose to lie down, rest on your side with a couple of pillows between your legs.

PAIN-RELIEVING DRUGS

If the above techniques don't provide sufficient comfort, you can go straight to the heavy hitters and use the various drugs available to help you physically. And we'll say it again—there's no shame in it whatsoever.

To determine what pain medication might be right for you, start by considering the side effects. Some drugs have very few, if any, whereas others can make you nauseous or potentially impact your baby's breathing at birth.

Although sedatives (which are drugs that calm, soothe and reduce irritability) won't take away pain, they are considered useful in reducing a woman's anxiety during early labor. They can also help an exhausted woman get some sleep. Sedatives can also help shorten the latent phase of labor, which is the longest stage.

Narcotics (a group of drugs that relieve pain and produce numbness) are known to "take the edge off" pain and dull it enough for a laboring woman to relax, but they do not take the pain away completely. This relaxation sometimes allows the cervix to dilate quicker, so ultimately narcotics may speed up labor.

Since narcotics and sedatives affect the entire body, and mother and baby may both experience their side effects. These include nausea, drowsiness and dizziness for Mom, and they can make Baby sleepy as well. These drugs are usually confined to the early part of labor and given in small doses so that they won't impact delivery. All side effects usually wear off in 2 to 4 hours.

Anesthesia (a substance that takes away pain and can induce deep sleep) is the most commonly used form of pain relief because it's very effective. There are two types: general and regional. General anesthesia puts the patient completely to sleep so he or she feels no pain at all. It can be effective within minutes, which is why it is primarily used for emergency C-sections. After the anesthesia wears off, the mother may feel groggy, disoriented and nauseous. Additionally, it creates a challenge for doctors, who must work to deliver the baby quickly before any anesthesia reaches him. Another risk of anesthesia is something we mentioned earlier. If the laboring woman's stomach contains any food or liquid, she could regurgitate it while unconscious and inhale the material into her lungs. Needless to say, this is dangerous, which is why hospitals tend to restrict food or drink by mouth. If time permits, antacids are usually given up to 30 minutes prior to the C-section to guard against this complication.

Regional anesthesia can block pain in a particular area of the body while allowing the patient to remain conscious. The great advantage here is that there is no effect on the baby and fewer side effects for Mom as well. The four kinds of regional anesthesia are:

1. Epidural block
2. Spinal block
3. Epidural/spinal block
4. Pudendal block

An epidural is pain medication that is administered through a tube inserted into the epidural space outside of the spinal cord in the lower back. Pain decreases in about 10 to 20 minutes, and the effect should last until delivery. Once the epidural needle is in place, the tube remains there during labor so that additional medication can be delivered if necessary.

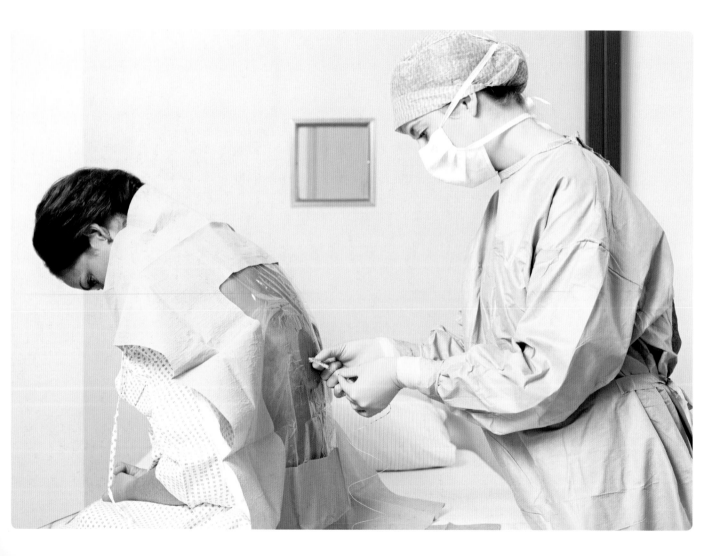

Depending on the dosage and type of medication, an epidural can cause numbness from the waist down, fully alleviating the pain of contractions and delivery (including pain in the vaginal and rectal area as well as pain from an episiotomy). The downside is that this blocks motor abilities, preventing the patient from moving around. It can also cut off the urge to push, though used in lower dosages the sensation of pressure remains.

Occasionally, epidurals can interfere with labor to the point where a C-section is needed. They also tend to cause the mother's blood pressure to drop, so that must be monitored carefully. And, finally, about 1 in 100 women experience severe headaches as a result of the epidural, sometimes even after they've been released from the hospital. This might necessitate a trip back to the hospital for treatment.

The spinal block involves injecting pain medication into the spinal fluid of the back. This numbs the lower half of the body and causes a loss of motor control from the waist down. Pain relief is immediate but lasts only 1 to 2 hours. A spinal block is usually administered only once during labor, so the goal is to delay its use until right before delivery. Possible side effects are the same as those associated with epidural anesthesia: lowered blood pressure and headaches.

Combined epidural and spinal anesthesia provides the benefits of the epidural block with the benefits of the spinal block. The epidural helps relieve pain throughout labor, while the spinal provides immediate relief. This medication is injected into the spinal fluid and into the space below the spinal cord, and it can relieve pain for up to 4 hours while allowing Mom to walk around.

In a pudendal block, pain medication is injected into the vaginal area to stop pain during the actual birth. Pain in the vagina and the area between the vaginal opening and anus is diminished, but the pain from contractions is not. This procedure can be used with episiotomies, especially when forceps or vacuums are needed. The pudendal block is considered relatively safe with few side effects.

Forceps are like a pair of tongs used to grasp a baby's head and help him through the birth canal. A forceps delivery may be used in special cases, such as when a mother has become too exhausted to complete the delivery without help or when the baby's heartbeat becomes dangerously irregular.

During a vacuum delivery, the practitioner places an object that looks like a plastic or metal cup on the baby's head and uses suction to help him through the birth canal. As in a forceps delivery, the practitioner opts for this in cases where Mom is utterly exhausted or there are signs of fetal distress.

The Second Stage of Labor

The second stage of labor usually brings big changes in the mood and in the pace and activities of labor. This stage begins once you've dilated to 10 cm, and it ends with the birth of your baby. Stage two lasts from 1 to 2 hours on average for first-time moms. For subsequent pregnancies, it might last less than an hour.

As you proceed through this stage, you're going to reach the expulsion phase, which is when you begin to feel a strong urge to push or bear down. In most cases, you're the one who signals this transition, either by telling your caregivers you want to push or reporting that you feel like you have to have a bowel movement. But—even if you say nothing—the expression on your face will probably give it away. The expulsion phase is also marked by the visible crowning of your baby's head at your pelvic rim—meaning that anyone who looks down there can see him starting to emerge. It's a very beautiful and odd sight at the same time. Discuss with your partner ahead of time whether he is permitted to film the miracle of your baby's birth.

Your pushing efforts, your position and the condition of the area between your anus and vagina all have an impact on your baby's birth. During this stage, you assume a more active role in the birth process. It's time for you to physically help and encourage your baby to come out into the world.

PUSHING DURING LABOR

The kind of pushing that's required to get baby through 10 cm of space is a "bearing down" kind of pushing, the kind associated with having a bowel movement. That may seem like an unpleasant comparison, but that's really what it's like!

POSITION DURING LABOR

Lying down at the onset of labor, or sometime soon after, and not getting up until after the baby has been born is an American phenomenon. Sitting upright, standing, kneeling or squatting for delivery is common in many other cultures—and with good reason. Moving into upright positions can facilitate a more natural labor using gravity to assist the baby's descent through the birth canal. Keep this in mind as you begin to think about how you want to manage your labor, but remember that it is your choice to make as long as all is proceeding safely.

MY PERINEUM?

As we discussed in Chapter 11, your perineum is a very special area. It's normal to cringe at the thought of an incision there (episiotomy), or, even worse, a spontaneous tear. Both situations require stitches, but episiotomies are often recommended to prevent unnecessary trauma to your body and to facilitate labor if natural progress has slowed down or ceased.

Although it has only just begun to be discussed and studied by the medical establishment, oiling and massaging the perineum is worth some consideration. Our great-great-grandmothers didn't need a study to believe that it was effective; it was routinely done prior to and during labor to thin out the tissue and make it supple and flexible enough for a baby to pass through without causing any tearing. Presently, nurse-midwives often place warm compresses at the perineum to help it stretch as the baby's head emerges.

CONGRATULATIONS, IT'S A . . .

It takes the coordination of your contractions, pushing and the baby's movements to get him to the final stretch of the birth canal. By the time he's there, you will probably have your second wind, energized by knowing that you will soon see and hold your baby. When his head reaches your vaginal opening, you will probably feel a stinging or burning sensation—but you may not feel it for long, since the pressure of his head will pinch and block the nerves down there. Your provider may administer regional anesthesia in anticipation of an episiotomy.

When the baby's head is delivered, it will mostly likely be face down, but the practitioner will turn it to the side, and then suction his mouth, nose and throat to remove any excess mucus. She or he may also check to make sure the umbilical cord is not wrapped around the baby's neck and remove it if it is. Your next two contractions will probably deliver one shoulder and then the other. The rest of your baby's body will slide out easily, probably followed by a flow of amniotic fluid. Congratulations! You are a mommy!

The Third Stage of Labor

WAIT, THERE'S MORE . . . AN ENCORE

Believe it or not, you're not finished working yet. The main objective of the third stage of labor is the delivery of the entire placenta with minimal blood loss. This stage begins about 5 to 10 minutes after the birth of your baby. Your caregiver will probably wait for your placenta to separate spontaneously from your uterine wall, evidenced by some blood and the further emergence of the umbilical cord. At that point, she or he will deliver your placenta. If the placenta doesn't separate from your uterine wall on its own, your caregiver can remove it manually by reaching in to get it.

Once the placenta has been delivered, your caregiver will examine it thoroughly to make sure no pieces of it have been left behind. Remnants of the placenta left in your uterus can cause postpartum hemorrhaging, or excessive bleeding (more on this later). Once both baby and placenta are safely out, your episiotomy incision or any lacerations can be repaired.

CESAREAN SECTIONS

A cesarean section, or C-section, is a surgical procedure during which small horizontal incisions are made in your abdomen and uterus through which your baby can be removed. This kind of delivery is performed when conditions exist that make vaginal delivery dangerous. Common conditions that require a C-section include a baby who is too large to pass through your pelvic area, signs that your baby's heart rate is abnormal, a baby who is lying sideways or whose feet or bottom are set to emerge first (breech birth), a labor that has been going on for too long without progressing or if you've had previous C-sections. This last one has come under scrutiny in previous years and there is a movement among some practitioners to attempt vaginal birth after C-sections.

Most C-sections are performed under epidural or spinal anesthesia, which (as described above) allows you to remain awake and hold your baby as soon as he is born. Nowadays, most hospitals will allow your partner to be with you during the operation.

If your C-section is necessitated by an emergency during labor—if, for example, your baby's heart rate becomes dangerously irregular—you may be put under general anesthesia and sleep through the procedure.

After a C-section, as after any surgery, you will need significant time to recover. You will experience pain around the incisions, but it can be relieved easily with pain medication. You will be encouraged to get up and move around early on. Laughing, sneezing and coughing may be uncomfortable, but holding your stomach will probably ease the pain. So, down comes the curtain on the big event. The cast of characters were right on cue, the newcomer made a spectacular debut and you—the star of the show—performed marvelously. Take a bow, for you deserve a standing ovation, and if you can't bow because of those C-section stitches, just pat yourself on the back. You were extraordinary!

Life after the Big Event

Now that the spotlights are off, the circus of caregivers have pretty much moved on and you have a new little person of your very own to care for, what can you expect? The next 6 weeks are considered the postpartum period, and it is during this time that your body will try to recover and snap back to its old, pre-pregnancy self. You will grapple with a number of physical and emotional adjustments all while taking care of a newborn baby. It can be an overwhelming time, so don't be too proud to allow family and friends to help out when they offer.

Many of the physical discomforts of the postpartum period can be alleviated by taking simple measures.

Your Uterus

Your uterus has to shrink back to its normal pre-pregnancy size, and this happens quite naturally. The material that made up your thick uterine wall breaks down and is absorbed by your body, and the cells themselves begin to shrink. You may experience "after-pains"—cramps caused by uterine contractions. Yes, more contractions, but they are necessary if you want to come close to fitting into your before-the-baby wardrobe. These contractions help reduce the size of your uterus as well as prevent hemorrhaging, and they last for just 2 to 3 days following birth. They are most severe during breast-feeding because your baby's sucking motions stimulate your pituitary gland, which in turn releases oxytocin—the hormone responsible for uterine contractions. If the discomfort of after-pains becomes intolerable, talk to your health-care provider about taking some mild pain medication.

Vaginal Discharge

You will notice a discharge after the birth of your baby, but it's not like your normal menstrual flow. It is called lochia (*LOH-kee-ah*) and is made up of blood cells, tissues from your uterine lining, cervical mucus and microorganisms. For the first 2 to 3 days following birth, lochia is dark red, then it turns pink and from about the third to the tenth day it's brown. The discharge may persist for an additional week or two after that and look yellowish or white. Lochia smells very much like a normal menstrual discharge, but if it has a foul smell, report this to your health-care provider as it may be a sign of infection.

Lochia can last up to 6 weeks, and while it continues, your cervix is still partially open, which means you are still at risk of an infection moving in through your vagina to your uterus. This is why doctors advise against using tampons, having sexual intercourse or even taking baths during the first 6 weeks after childbirth.

If you are not nursing your baby, you can expect your regular menstrual flow to recommence about 6 to 8 weeks after the birth. If you are nursing, you may not menstruate until you've partially or completely stopped breast-feeding. But be sure to use birth control during this time because even though you may not be getting your period, you can still become pregnant. That is worth saying again. Be very careful to guard against unwanted pregnancies. The fact that you aren't menstruating doesn't mean you can't get pregnant!

Postpartum Hemorrhaging

Although not a normal postpartum occurrence, excessive bleeding after the birth of a baby takes the lives of too many black women. That's right. We have the highest risk for maternal mortality—and one of the reasons is excessive bleeding after childbirth. Some risk factors associated with postpartum hemorrhaging are delivering a very large baby, having part of the placenta left attached to the uterine wall, being obese and having a uterus that doesn't contract effectively. The good news is doctors are trained to counteract these risks with preventive measures prior to and during childbirth. Be sure to talk with your health-care professional about these risks.

Perineal Pain

During the postpartum period, you will probably feel some pain in your perineum, vaginal and anal areas. The soft tissue surrounding your vagina and anus are swollen and bruised from all it has been through. If you had an episiotomy or tore naturally and needed stitches, those can contribute to your discomfort. Applying ice packs or cotton balls soaked in witch hazel to the area is your best form of relief. Walking helps the healing process, too, because it stimulates circulation.

Fear of Urinating & Bowel Movements

We don't blame you for feeling apprehensive about relieving yourself after childbirth. Urinating can be painful as the liquid passes over the cuts and bruises of your perineum. Pouring water over the area from a water bottle as you pee may help reduce the sting.

Your bowels may be sluggish because of your decreased abdominal muscle tone. That, coupled with the fear of tearing out your stitches if you bear down, may make you want to avoid bowel movements altogether—but of course that's one of the worst things you can do. Reluctance to relieve yourself can lead to constipation (hard stools)—making it even more painful when you do finally have a bowel movement. It all has to come out sometime! To ensure bowel health and easier bathroom sessions, eat plenty of fruit, whole grains and fresh veggies, and drink plenty of liquids.

Tender Breasts

Whether you feed your baby via breast or bottle, your breasts may be tender and sore for a while. Your body is naturally producing milk at first, engorging your breasts. If you do nurse, the pain will diminish with feedings. Make sure your newborn attaches completely and avoid drying soaps and alcohol-based products to keep your nipples moist and supple.

If you're not breast-feeding, you may want your milk to dry out naturally. Wearing a snug fitting support bra and applying ice packs to breasts can ease pain. Don't express the milk because that signals your body to make more. Avoid running warm water over your breasts and try not to stimulate your nipples in any way, as these things will only increase your milk production.

Your breasts may remain engorged for about 4 days after delivery. If your milk doesn't begin to dry up after that or if pain persists and is accompanied by fever or hardened areas in your breasts, call your doctor. These symptoms may indicate a plugged duct or infection.

Loose Abdomen

The baby's gone but the stomach's still there, all loose and flabby. Your abdomen did a lot of stretching, and it's logical that it may take some time to get it back to its old shape. Fortunately, this area responds well to exercise, and with a little effort on your part, you should be back to normal within 2 to 3 months. So don't get discouraged and let yourself go. Yes, you have a new baby to care for, but you still have *you* to care for, too.

Weight Loss

You can expect to lose about 10 to 12 pounds as a direct result of the birth of your baby, the removal of your placenta and the loss of amniotic fluid. Just urinating during the first few days after birth may net an additional 5-pound loss. If you were successful at limiting the amount of weight you gained during pregnancy to 25 to 30 pounds, it should only take you a couple of months to return to your pre-pregnancy weight. But even if you gained more weight than necessary, don't get discouraged. Once you receive the OK from your doctor, commit yourself to a sensible exercise regimen and a healthy, well-balanced diet, and you'll reach your goal.

Postpartum Blues and Sometimes Depression

It's common for new mothers to experience mood swings, ambivalent feelings toward motherhood and even mild depression. A little patience from your loved ones—and yourself—can go a long way now.

Remember that you have a lot to adjust to. You are still physically worn out from pregnancy and childbirth, to say nothing of the sleep deprivation you are experiencing now. And your hormones are still out of balance. Try to listen to your body, get as much rest and sleep as you can and be patient with yourself.

Don't underestimate the havoc sleep deprivation can cause, not just to your body, but to your emotions, as well. "I'm tired all the time" is probably the biggest complaint we hear from postpartum women. Again—understand that this is temporary. Believe it or not, your baby will soon mature to a point where he can sleep through the night.

Although it may not seem like it during a 3:00 a.m. feeding, newborns spend a lot of time sleeping. These frequent naps provide you with great opportunities to sleep or rest as well, which in turn will help your emotional stability.

If you're feeling blue, remember that this is normal and probably temporary. There's nothing wrong with you just because you are not 100 percent happy and giddy in love with your new life. Many women are not. It will pass.

But if your "blue period" lasts longer than a couple of weeks and you feel you may be falling into a depression, speak to your health-care provider. Postpartum depression affects approximately 10 to 15 percent of women, and black women have an increased risk for it. Although you may not want to speak to anyone about your feelings, you have to resist the tendency to avoid seeking help. If you are depressed, your relationships with the people around you are more than likely affected by your emotional state, which includes the newest member of your family. Infants are highly sensitive to the people around them. Depression in new mothers can deprive babies of the very important mother-baby bond, and, as a consequence, impair the infant developmental process. So, if you can't bring yourself to seek help right now for yourself, let that little face who wants nothing more than your unconditional love and attention be your motivation. You may just need some professional assistance for a while, and there are a number of organizations and agencies specializing in mental-health care for black people, such as these:

- The Association of Black Psychologists: www.abpsi.org
- Black Mental Health Alliance: www.blackmentalhealth.com
- National Organization for People of Color Against Suicide: www.nopcas.org
- Black Psychiatrists of America: www.bpaincpsych.org
- National Association of Black Social Workers: www.nabsw.org

So maybe it does seem a little unfair. For the last 9 months you've had to maintain the perfect environment for your unborn baby, then you had to endure the pain of labor and birth, and still, your body and mind are compromised in various ways—to say nothing of your time and energy. But you have done something no one else on this earth could do: you've become the mother of your child. I'm sure you agree that it was well worth the effort! My sixteen-year-old son recently mailed (mailed!) me a letter from school. Here is an unedited excerpt, and I promise you it is the real thing:

Dear Mom,

I love you, and you inspire me so much. Without you I'd be nothing, and I am so grateful that you raised me. I know what a struggle it must have been to raise me alone for so long. We have a bond that can never be broken, and that is really special to me. I still remember those days of you hustling alone just to make me the happiest kid in the world.

I have probably embarrassed the living daylights out of him by sharing this, but for you, my sister, it is worth it. You, too, will come to know a love that is beyond words. And all of the physical pain and other compromises will pale in comparison. Trust me, you'll see.

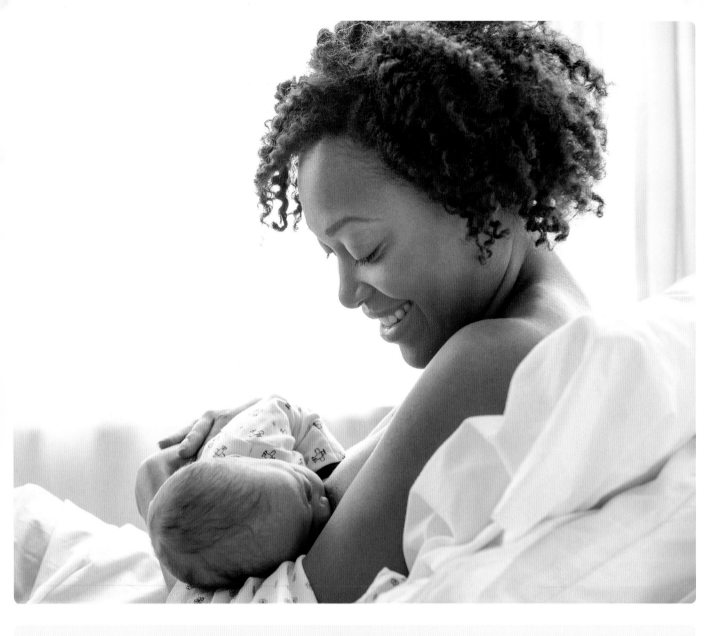

— CHAPTER 15 —

Your Newborn

The experience of unconditional love starts here for most women. Once your baby is placed in your arms, with little time to even take a good look at her, you're in love. She's yours, and you love that. It doesn't even matter that her head is cone-shaped from pressing on your cervix for hours or that she's covered in a greasy, cheese-like substance. You hold her, kiss her and experience such a wonderful and loving feeling.

But once you do get a chance to really check her out, you'll notice that newborns are a little different from the one-month-old babies we're used to seeing on TV. Here are some typical first impressions we see in newly born babies.

Baby's Skin

Most babies, regardless if they're black or white, look the same immediately after delivery. The newborn's skin color is usually very light, which can cause you and that mahogany-brown man of yours to do a double take. A newborn is also usually covered with the greasy, grayish-white vernix caseosa that we discussed in prior chapters. The vernix was needed to protect your baby's skin during her long residency in amniotic fluid. Bluish-black spots, medically known as Mongolian spots, may also be present on her lower back or buttocks. They're especially common in black babies. These spots pose no harm or threat and will most likely disappear during early childhood. A newborn's skin may also peel a lot right around her hands and feet, but that should stop a few days after birth. Even with all of that going on, babies are inherently beautiful, that's why we find it hard to put down the camera.

Baby's Head

If you deliver vaginally, your newborn's head may be lopsided or pointed as a result of her trip through the birth canal. But relax. It'll eventually take on a more normal shape. On the top of the head is the baby's soft spot, called the fontanelle (*fahn-teh-NEHL*). Many of us remember picking up newborn babies when we were younger and everybody warning us to be careful of the baby's soft spot. This area is soft because the bones of the newborn's skull have not joined together yet, which should happen by the time she's 18 months to 24 months old.

Baby's Eyes

Your newborn's eyelids may look puffy and swollen. She may also squint a lot and her eyes may even look slightly crossed. These conditions are not permanent and should clear up in the first few weeks of life. If they do not, or if you're just concerned, discuss it with your pediatrician.

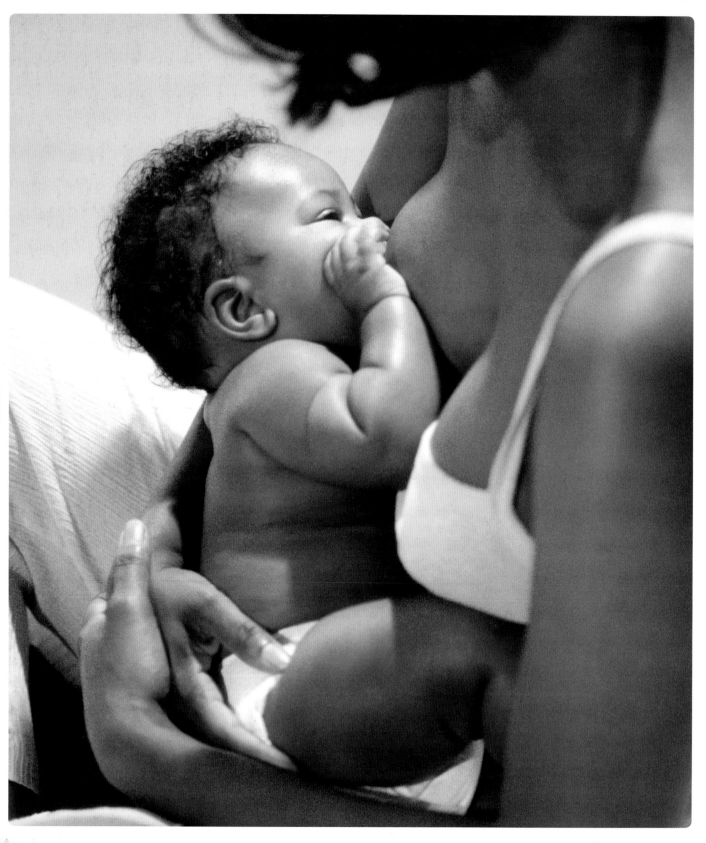

Baby's Hair

A newborn may have thick hair or thin hair, and it could be curly or straight. She may even have almost no hair at all. Whatever it is, just don't refer to it as "good hair" or "bad hair," and don't allow anybody else to do that, either—there's no such thing! You're too smart and strong to allow yourself to fall for that nonsense now. Plus, you are now raising a beautiful black baby whose self-esteem and self-awareness, whether positive or negative, is dependent largely upon you, a beautiful black woman. So let's just get over it!

What a wonderful challenge you have ahead of you. You truly have an opportunity for improving the world. Your baby has unlimited potential. But before you can give him all that he needs to realize his potential, your needs must be attended to.

In many ways parenting is synonymous with giving; however, you can't give what you don't have. That's why it's vital for you as a parent to take the time, effort, money and so on to fulfill your own basic needs so you can adequately fulfill the needs of your children. You must have a reservoir of patience, for example, so that you can show and give your children patience. You need to have a good reserve of love, respect and acceptance to be able to shower those qualities on your children and certainly before you can imbed them in their own character.

More powerful than any amount of money that you can possess is a positive attitude. So be proud! Be proud that you're black and be proud of the fact that you just may be growing the next social scientist who will teach us how to put an end to racism or the next physician who will discover how to destroy cancer cells without harming the rest of the body. Obstacles? Yes, there will be some, but nothing you can't handle. The real challenge is seeing the blessing in them. Coping with complications is inherent for us, generally speaking. It makes us stronger and teaches us how to persevere.

As you proceed on your journey to motherhood, remember that the nurturing and care your baby needs begins now. Your unborn baby's source of sustenance is you—nothing else and no one else. If you want to capitalize on all of her potential, make sure you feed her nervous system and all of her other life-support systems with the nutrients she needs to thrive.

Sustenance for your baby comes in the form of love as well. Surround yourself with love and warmth, and that'll be the quality of life your child will come to know.

Enjoy this special time in your life and the rewards you will continue to receive from that beautiful, little brown face!

Appendix A

A Positive Approach to Government Assistance

Your family is growing, your belly is growing, but your wallet remains the same. Yes, babies are our gifts in life, but they come with many expenses. You may be wondering where the extra money will come from, especially if you are living on a tight budget already.

Federal and state benefit programs are available for eligible individuals and families in need of a safe place to live or adequate food or health care, and we encourage you to look into any program you might qualify for. Although sometimes there is a negative stigma associated with needing public assistance, there is nothing wrong with asking for and accepting help. No one should go hungry or homeless in one of the richest countries in the world.

The website www.benefits.gov provides a comprehensive rundown of thousands of programs available from federal and state agencies. You can also walk into your local Department of Social Services for direct help. (Find the nearest location by searching online or at your local library.)

Once you've determined which programs might work for you, how can you start the ball rolling? Accepting aid from the government is a two-part process. Your first step is to contact the local agencies that administer the benefit programs. Through some strategic googling, you may find this is as simple as filling out some web-based application. (If you don't have a computer at home, you can probably find one at your local library.) Alternatively, you might be able to apply by mail, fax or in person at a local agency office. However you choose to proceed, though, make sure you adhere precisely to the application guidelines so as not to waste your precious time on bureaucracy.

Whatever aid you're applying for, you'll certainly have to prove your eligibility, so be prepared with whatever documentation is required (birth certificate, social security card, proof of residency, etc.). The process may not be easy, but it is worthwhile for you and your family.

Let's say you've jumped through all of the hoops and you have qualified for assistance. The checks come in. Life is moving along—you are getting what you and your family need and deserve. So what's the second step we mentioned? The second big step is just as important as the first, and that is to develop a realistic plan for leaving public assistance behind.

We believe that your ultimate financial independence is as critical to your family's well-being as ample food and a roof over your head. Without a plan for eventually walking away from government assistance, you increase your chances of permanent helplessness and entrapment in a cycle of poverty and substandard living conditions.

In addition to your plans for getting onto and off of public assistance, it's important to expose yourself and your family to people and experiences outside of the culture of poverty on a regular basis. Try visiting friends or relatives on Saturday or Sunday afternoons. Seek out strong family members, develop support systems and look for inspiring teachers or clergy. Children's museums, libraries, learning centers and bookstores are positive environments that can encourage and inspire you and your child. Yes, these may require some planning and travel, but the effort is sure to prove worthwhile.

More important than the influence of others is summoning up a strong sense of personal motivation. You will need to develop or strengthen skills and values that will inspire you and help you advance yourself. Apply your knowledge and experience and use your support systems. When preparing for a job interview, perhaps a friend can help you craft your résumé or put together the right outfit to impress the interviewer. If you are facing an afternoon of waiting in line at a government agency, ask a loved one to babysit so you can use the waiting time to read, think and recharge your batteries. These experiences are frustrating enough without the children working your nerves.

Never think of the social programs you are involved with as ends in themselves; think of them as the means to a greater end. That being the case, you have to bring your A-game to every experience. For example, if you are enrolled in a job-training program (a very good idea if you are unemployed), punctuality and regular participation are important. If you are receiving monetary assistance, spend those checks wisely, in ways that affect the future of your family and not just their momentary desires. And throughout the process keep in mind that your persistence and motivation will help you avoid perpetual poverty. When it all seems hard to handle, take comfort from the fact that being a good role model is the best gift you can give your kids.

Appendix B

Prenatal Appointment Schedule Worksheet

Use this form to track the important information that gets discussed during your prenatal visits. Make a copy of it every month, and jot down the questions you want to ask your health-care provider during any of your upcoming appointments. Be prepared to write down answers and some of your personal data that gets collected, such as your weight and blood pressure.

WORKSHEET

Prenatal Appointment Schedule

Date & Time: _____   Weeks Pregnant: _____

Pre-pregnancy Weight: _____   Current Weight: _____

Last Menstrual Period (LMP): _____   Blood Pressure: _____

Caregiver Comments: _____

What that means to me: _____

My Question: _____

Response:

My Question: _____

Response:

Notes:

Appendix C

A Quick Look at How Each State Supports Pregnant and New Parents

Below is a snapshot of what each state offers pregnant women and new parents beyond federal mandates. The information is not all-encompassing, because even though a state may offer provisions beyond federal law, conditions are more than likely attached to the entitlement.

Private workers are individuals who work in nongovernmental, privately owned companies. State workers are individuals who work for the government in federal, state, provincial or municipal positions.

State Offers	More than the Federal FMLA		More than the Nursing Mothers' Workplace Rights		Maternity Leave		Use of Sick Time		Nothing Beyond Federal Laws	
	Private Workers	State Workers	Private Workers	State Workers	Private Workers	State Worker	Private Workers	State Workers	Private Workers	State Workers
Alabama									X	X
Alaska		X							X	
Arizona		X								
Arkansas			X	X						
California	X	X	X	X	X	X	X	X		
Colorado		X	X	X				X		
Connecticut	X	X	X	X	X	X	X			
Delaware								X	X	
District of Columbia	X	X	X	X			X	X		
Florida		X							X	
Georgia									X	X
Hawaii	X	X			X	X	X	X		
Idaho									X	X
Illinois		X	X	X		X				
Indiana			X	X						
Iowa					X	X				
Kansas									X	X

(continued)

State Offers	More than the Federal FMLA		More than the Nursing Mothers' Workplace Rights		Maternity Leave		Use of Sick Time		Nothing Beyond Federal Laws	
	Private Workers	State Workers	Private Workers	State Workers	Private Workers	State Worker	Private Workers	State Workers	Private Workers	State Workers
Kentucky						X			X	
Louisiana					X	X				
Maine	X	X	X	X			X	X		
Maryland							X	X		
Massachusetts					X	X				
Michigan										
Minnesota	X	X	X	X						
Mississippi									X	X
Missouri								X	X	
Montana				X	X	X				
Nebraska									X	X
Nevada									X	X
New Hampshire					X	X				
New Jersey	X	X			X	X		X		
New Mexico			X	X						
New York		X	X	X	X	X				
North Carolina									X	X
North Dakota									X	X
Ohio		X				X		X	X	
Oklahoma									X	X
Oregon	X	X	X	X			X	X		
Pennsylvania		X							X	
Rhode Island	X	X	X	X	X	X		X		
South Carolina								X	X	
South Dakota									X	X
Tennessee	X	X	X	X				X		
Texas		X						X	X	
Utah								X	X	
Vermont	X	X	X	X						
Virginia						X			X	
Washington	X	X			X		X	X		
West Virginia									X	X
Wisconsin	X	X					X	X		
Wyoming									X	X

Acknowledgments

First and foremost I would like to thank Dr. Suzanne Greenidge-Hewitt. I couldn't have done it without her, and, quite honestly, I would never have tried to do so. She is the best coauthor, the coolest friend and such a skilled doctor. The next most sincere appreciation goes to Laura Ross, our editor and publishing consultant. Her dedicated interest in this book and belief in Suzanne and me is what led us to the good people at Page Street Publishing. And the good people at Page Street Publishing are Will Kiester, publisher, to whom we are indebted for sharing our vision of getting this book into the hands of the women who need it, and Marissa Giambelluca, acquisitions and editorial manager. We would be remiss if we didn't acknowledge the Page Street design team along with everyone else at Page Street who had a hand in getting this book published.

I must also thank the best husband in the world, Bernard, for his sheer love and support for me, as well as my son, Brendon, and daughters Annelise, Mia and Sara, the beautiful brown faces I come home to every day. This book is dedicated to the other little brown faces in the schools across this country who have inspired me to do all I can to help them thrive and live the high-quality lives we all deserve.

I thank my sister, Pat Braswell, for always being there for me, as well as Alexis Caudle, a talented graphic designer and overall supporter of *Black, Pregnant and Loving It*. I would also like to thank Dr. Sumayah Jamal for sharing her expertise in the dermatologic care of women of color. Many thanks go to Leslie Louard-Davis, a longtime friend and advocate. It's so precious to have people like Leslie in my life who will do whatever they can to promote a friend's cause. Harriet Roy, Susan Saban, Renee Allen-Walker, Amy Goldstein and Heather Palmore are all good friends who fit the bill.

—Yvette Allen-Campbell

This book is more than 20 years in the making. It is a labor of love and a gift for wonderful, beautiful, black pregnant women. It is also an expression of gratitude to all those I have served and learned from during my 26 years as an obstetrician/gynecologist. Special thanks and praise to my coauthor Yvette Allen-Campbell, who originated and championed this project before there was ever a word on paper. She has been the backbone of *Black, Pregnant and Loving It*. Yvette found me during my OB/GYN residency at Harlem Hospital in New York City and convinced me of a special need for this book. She is a great friend, my cheerleader and a wonderful coauthor. I look forward to our next book together.

The book benefited greatly from Laura Ross's literary acumen, and I am grateful to her for her patience, encouragement and support while producing the wonderful proposal that led us to the hands of our publisher, Page Street. I would like to thank Page Street Publishing's acquisitions and editorial manager Marissa Giambelluca and publisher William Kiester for seeing the need for this book.

(continued)

Special acknowledgements are needed for James Bernasko, professor of maternal fetal medicine at Stony Brook University Hospital, for helping us with his expertise, and to my OB/GYN colleagues and longtime friends Evelyn Minaya, MD; Gail McDonald, MD; Deborah White, MD; and Paige Long, MD; for reviewing, encouraging and being in my corner for many years.

To my forever cheerleaders—my patients and my staff at Woman to Woman OB/GYN Medical Group. I thank you for giving me continued support every day and the flexibility to do this. My office manager, Nedine Tarby-Richards, is always in my corner, working every angle of my practice and medical career to ensure my success.

Heartfelt thanks to chef Denzil Richards of New York City (husband of Nedine Tarby-Richards), who provided the wonderful dishes to add the special culinary touch to this book.

Finally, I would like to thank my family. I dedicate my first published book to my grandparents Edna and Lawson Greenidge, the two people who first supported my dream of becoming a doctor. Dr. Cynthia Degazon, my aunt, who gives me daily support and guidance through all my endeavors. Many thanks to my parents, Norma Armstrong, Thomas Armstrong (stepfather) and Granville Straker. I am thankful to all of my siblings for their unwavering and unconditional support. Last, but not least, many thanks to my wonderful firefighter husband of 29 years, Marstus Hewitt, and my children, Makaelah and Jaelee, for providing love and the constant inspiration for me to be my best for them. I especially look forward to the day this book will provide guidance for my future grandchildren.

—Dr. Suzanne Greenidge-Hewitt

About the Authors

Yvette Allen-Campbell is a leader in the field of education. Over the past 30 years, she has worked for children as a teacher of the speech and hearing impaired, supervisor of speech and language therapists, assistant principal, principal and now central office supervisor. She believes leadership can evolve naturally to those who are well balanced enough to cultivate relationships with others who want to follow. She relishes the dynamics of a team of talented, motivated individuals who want to work hard toward a common goal. She also sincerely believes that we must not only commit to teaching children subjects like science or a curriculum, we must also desire to connect with children. She is known for proclaiming that to educate, really educate, children, teachers must first have a sincere and respectful desire to know what their students already know and how they came to know it. Then the process of meshing the new with the old can be facilitated optimally.

Suzanne Greenidge-Hewitt, MD, is a board-certified obstetrician/gynecologist who has been practicing for 26 years. She is the founder, CEO and medical director of Woman to Woman OB/GYN, a top-ranked New York–based comprehensive medical center. She specializes in laparoscopic and robotic gynecologic surgery and is an avid spokesperson for women's reproductive health. Dr. Greenidge-Hewitt serves as a senior attending at St John's Riverside Hospital, New York-Presbyterian/Lawrence Hospital, and St Joseph's Medical Center. From 1994 to 2015, she was an assistant clinical professor and clinical attending at New York Columbia Presbyterian Hospital.

As an African American woman and mother, Dr. Greenidge-Hewitt deeply understands the hopes, dreams and aspirations that black mothers have from conception and their fears and anxieties about raising a healthy, balanced child in a challenging American landscape. She speaks to these issues with authority but also with uncommon compassion for mothers. Being able to safely deliver babies has been her passion since the age of 10. Having witnessed her own mother's trauma following a missed diagnosis during prenatal care with her sister, Dr. Greenidge-Hewitt has deep wisdom to share about the importance of effective prenatal care, particularly for black women.

Dr. Greenidge-Hewitt is especially proud of being the mother of two beautiful, vivacious daughters—the next generation of black women.

Index

orgasms, 84
oxytocin, 199

p

pain
  anesthesia, 193–194
  aromatherapy for, 192
  breasts, 92, 201
  causes of, 190–191
  cervical dilation and, 190
  compresses for, 192
  contractions and, 190
  drug-free management of,
      191–193
  massage for, 82–83, 178, 192
  medications for, 141, 188, 193–195
  meditation for, 191
  music for, 192
  narcotics for, 193
  perineum, 200
  pubic area, 174
  repositioning for, 192
  touch for, 192
  visualization for, 192
  water births and, 139
papaya, in All-Fruit Fruit Salad
      with Raspberry Syrup, 50
partial previa, 73
partners
  communication and, 142–143, 151
  counseling and, 126–127
  C-sections and, 198
  delivery and, 177
  eighth month, 170–171
  emotional stability with, 170–171
  fifth month, 142–143
  filming and, 184, 196
  first month and, 101
  fourth month, 126–127
  hospital bag for, 184–185
  money and, 162
  ninth month, 177
  participation of, 118–119
  physical changes and, 151
  second month and, 109–110
  seventh month, 162
  sixth month, 151
  third month, 118–119
paternity leave, 30
peak flow meter, 63
pears, in All-Fruit Fruit Salad with
      Raspberry Syrup, 50

peas, in Potato Salad, 49
perinatologists, 23
perineum
  episiotomies, 21, 197
  massaging, 163, 197
  pain, 200
  postpartum period and, 200
  urination and, 200
  stretching, 163
pertussis, 160
phychotherapy, 94
physical appearance
  first month, 89
  second month, 104–107
  third month, 113
  fourth month, 121
  fifth month, 130
  sixth month, 145
  seventh month, 154
  eighth month, 165
  ninth month, 173
physical examinations, 98
physical symptoms
  first month, 89–94
  second month, 107–108
  third month, 114–115
  fourth month, 122–123
  fifth month, 131–132
  sixth month, 147
  seventh month, 155–158
  eighth month, 166–169
  ninth month, 173–175
pineapple, in All-Fruit Fruit Salad
      with Raspberry Syrup, 50
placenta
  blood flow to, 77
  chorionic villi, 116
  cigarettes and, 78
  cocaine and, 79
  delivery of, 197–198
  development of, 123
  fibroids, 76
  folic acid and, 37
  function of, 123–124
  hypertension and, 55
  placenta abruptio, 73, 74
  placenta accreta, 74, 75
  placenta increta, 74, 75
  placenta percreta, 74, 75
  placenta previa, 73
  postpartum hemorrhaging and,
      200
  third-trimester bleeding and,
      73–75

umbilical cord, 117
pork loin, in sautéed Sesame Seed
      Medallion Pork Loin in
      Honey Glaze Sauce, 47
positions
  for delivery, 22
  for labor, 192, 196
  for sex, 84
  for sleep, 55, 175
  for supine hypotensive
      syndrome, 158
postpartum period
  abdominal looseness, 201
  ambivalence, 201
  bowel movements and, 200
  breast tenderness, 201
  contractions and, 199
  depression, 201–203
  discharge, 199
  hemorrhaging, 200
  menstruation and, 200
  perineal pain, 200
  pregnancy and, 200
  sleep, 202
  urination and, 200
  uterus and, 199
  vaginal discharge, 199
  weight and, 201
potatoes
  Brown Stew Chicken, 44
  Potato Salad, 49
preeclampsia
  calcium and, 38
  chronic hypertension and, 59
  ethnicity and, 53
  gestational hypertension and,
      58
  "Jamie" and, 60
  protein and, 100
  superimposed on chronic
      hypertension, 59–60
  symptoms of, 59
  treatment for, 59
Pregnancy Discrimination Act
      (1978), 27
"pregnancy haze," 165
prenatal screening tests, 117
preterm births
  definition of, 68
  NICU and, 159
  prevention of, 68
  surfactant, 150
  treatment for, 70
preterm labor